The Unity
Guide to Healing

Compiled by Connie Fillmore

Contents

The Spirit and the Life 5

The Great Healer 13

God's Greatest Gift 19

The Power of the Word 29

Man's Creative Thought 37

Contacting the Source 47

Mental Cause Revealed 61

Live Wisely and Well 73

The Body Temple 83

The Myth of Aging 93

The Way to Healing 99

Treatments for Specific Disorders 109

Two Healing Testimonies 117

References 121

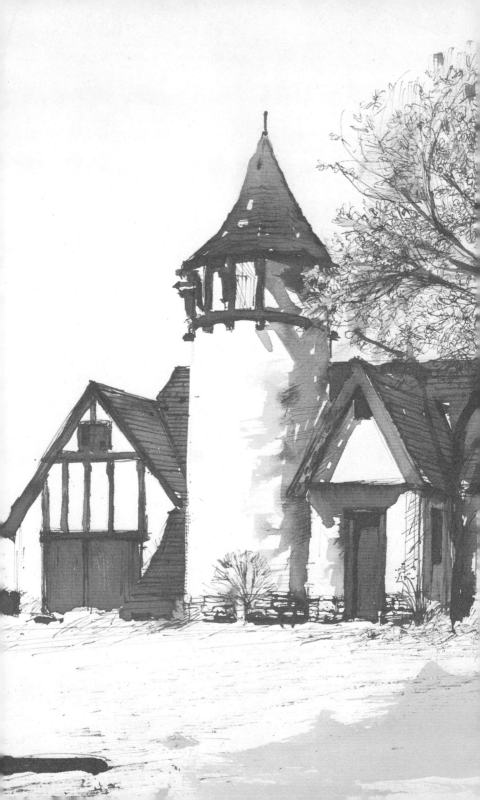

The Spirit and the Life

All our happiness, all our health and power, come from God. They flow in an unbroken stream from the fountainhead into the very center of our being, and radiate from center to circumference. God is the one perfect life flowing through us. God is the one pure substance out of which our organism is formed. God is the power that gives us motive power; the strength that holds us upright and allows us to exercise our members; the wisdom that gives us intelligence in every cell of our organism, every thought of our mind. God is the only reality of us.

God does not exercise power. God *is* all-present and all-quiet power from which man generates his own power.

God does not manifest intelligence. God *is* that unobtrusive knowing in everyone which, when acknowledged, flashes forth into intelligence.

God is not matter, nor confined in any way to the idea of substance termed matter. God is substance, but this does not mean matter, because matter is formed, while God is the formless. This substance which God is lies back of all matter and all forms. It is that which is the basis of all form, yet enters not into any form as finality. It cannot be seen, tasted, or touched.

Energy Distinct from Matter

God is Spirit, and Spirit is the very essence of the ether in which we live, move, and have our being. Spirit is life or living substance considered independently of corporeal existence; it is an intelligence apart from any physical organization or embodiment. Spirit is vital essence, force, or energy, as distinct from matter; it is the intelligent, immaterial, and immortal part of man.

5

Life is the activity of God. It is principle, the animating force, the every-where-present potential of livingness. It is a principle that is made manifest in the living. Life cannot be analyzed by the senses. It is beyond their grasp; hence it must be cognized by Spirit. Life is not involved in time; it has no beginning and no end. Individually, however, life is that universal force projected into a particular form and manner of expression, that is, man. Spirit is all. Where would you draw the line between Spirit and the material, when there is no evidence that God has placed such boundaries? We see Spirit manifesting in the flesh, in the centers of consciousness, and in the organs of the body as expressions of energy and substance. All life is divine; all life is the breath of God. All life is God made manifest, and the manifestation varies according to the degree in which God, the breath of life, comes forth into visibility through the various forms. Man is the fullest, highest form of God manifested as life.

We read that "in the beginning" this mysterious something, which we cannot see, feel, or handle but which is plainly stated to be the "breath of God," was breathed into clay man and "man became a living being." God created a perfect spiritual man in the beginning. Surely such a man would live in a perfect body. The life of every being is the "breath of God," today, just as it always has been. Life never changes, but exists eternal in every child of God. Neither the soul of man nor the body of man has life in itself. Both are made alive and kept alive momently by the Spirit that is God pervading and permeating them.

Boundless energy and enthusiasm for life are inherent in each of us, as evidenced by the nature of the child. Few of us demonstrate this vitality throughout our lives, and yet we envy and admire those who do. The difference is not in the amount of energy possessed, but in the way the energy is used. Even the most tired and listless person has what amounts to a dynamo of energy hidden in the least little cell of his body. He does not seem to have energy because he does not use the energy he has. He does not let this life, which is the life of God within him, express itself through him. If the small child bounds with energy, so should we! The life of God in us is unchanging; it is no different in a child than it is in an adult. There is no reason for us to lose the feeling of limitless energy and enthusiasm. There is within us a strong, compelling will to live. With every breath, we affirm life. Nothing can defeat the life within us, for it is of God; it is without beginning or end; it is free and pure and perfect; it cannot be weakened by the appearance of disease. It is powerful, perfect, ceaseless, changeless—and it is within us.

God is the health of His people. He was never sick a day; He is the source of life and health and joy. God wills that we express His "image" and "likeness," in which we were created. The will to be well comes from Him, and the Spirit that does the healing work is not far from us. Healing does not depend on externals. God is mighty in the midst of us to vitalize, renew, and heal us. What we cannot do through our own efforts, through an act of will, God does easily and effortlessly in and through us. We do not have to strain after health, for God is with us as perfect health at all times.

The Urge toward Perfection

Because man is a spiritual being, he is forever the focus of a spiritual power that works to manifest life in perfect health and harmony and abundance. "It is your Father's good pleasure to give you the kingdom." It is the life of God through which the life of man is forever biased on the side of health and healing.

A state of health is a condition of wholeness, completeness, entireness. Men are creations in God's image, and healing is merely the bringing forth of the natural, perfect Christ that exists within every man. Health is the natural state of man. The word to *heal* comes from the Saxon *helian:* to cover, to conceal, to be made whole. Thus a healthy man is a whole one, one who lives and functions just as his Creator intended him to. Health is fundamental in Being and health is man's divine birthright. It is the orderly state of existence, and man must learn to use the knowledge of this truth to sustain the consciousness of health.

Inherent Healing Power

We find that there is an omnipresent principle of health pervading all living things. Health, real health, is from within and does not have to be manufactured in the without. Health is the very essence of Being and is as universal and enduring as God. This spirit of wholeness is called the Holy Spirit in the New Testament. In classical mythology it is called Hygeia. Modern medical men refer to it as the restorative power of nature. It has been recognized by savage and civilized alike in every land and age. It has many names, and they all identify it as a universal urge toward perfection in man and toward keeping things going regardless of any interfering force. No method of healing can create new cells within the body of a living organism; only the creative forces in the body can do this. The organism tends to maintain itself if it is not interfered with. The creative forces are self-sufficient. They need no help. They just need "no interference," or the removal of obstructions that impede their natural action. To clear the way for the innate, creative forces, then, is the true purpose of healing agencies. No matter what course may be pursued or how the healing law is employed, the goal is to establish wholeness, to evoke the perfect activity of the life force which renews, rebuilds, and sustains the body. Only one healing power exists, whether evoked by methods of physician, witch doctor, or metaphysician. The goal is not surgery for its own sake, or medication for its own sake, or even prayer for its own sake. These methods are employed to release the inherent healing power and to restore the body to its normal condition of health. Whether the life principle's energy is activated by meditation or by medication makes no difference. Health is more life. Drugs cannot of themselves give life. Travel and change of scene, so often resorted to in illness of mind and body, will not give life except insofar as they tend to relax the tense, rigid mind and body of man and permit God to flow in to fill the lack. We do not have to beseech God. Life more abundant rushes into the minds and bodies of men, as air does into a vacuum, the moment they learn how consciously to relax and, turning toward God, let it.

Inner, Energetic Life

The healing of a sick body depends upon the life force that is within the body. Something may be done by outer means to assist and encourage this indwelling healing power, but this assistance by itself cannot heal or build up a broken, weak body. A surgeon can set a broken bone, but he must depend upon the inner life force of the body to knit the parts together. Jesus did not produce the healing which He introduced into the world. Healing comes when the soul contacts God. The Physician does not bestow health; He joins us to health. The natural laws that create and sustain the body are really divine laws, and when man asks for the intervention of God in restoring health, he is calling into action the natural forces of his being. These laws are exact and undeviating; results are unfailing if one can make connection with the natural life forces and allow them to work through him. The law of healing is a demonstrable principle, as effective today as it was two thousand years ago in the time of Jesus. It manifests for each individual according to his consciousness. Behind every personal mind is the recreative Mind. God-Mind not only can restore and heal but can establish us in the consciousness of permanent health.

We may be relieved of bodily ills and yet not be healed. A healing is more than a bringing of flesh and bone and nerve and blood to a state of soundness and regular action. Healing does not stop at bringing back the vigor of body enjoyed in youth, when life was a joy of coordinating muscles and rhythmic functionings. It does not stop at a restoration to the state of organic freedom which was known in childhood.

Reaching the Source

To be healed is to be restored to the original state of being. Healed, we shall live in perfection. Healing is the frictionless relationship of life and environment. It is found where life is found: in God. Healing begins where life begins: in God. We must go to God in order to be healed. If we cannot reach God, we can only temporarily alleviate symptoms. No true healing is done without reaching back to the Source.

The source of healing is quickened life energy in the body. Jesus Christ healed by revitalizing the life energy that already existed in His students, yet had become sluggish and unused through error thought. When we worship God in His way, we are vitalized all at once; there is no other way to get real, permanent life. This life is not available from outer sources. The life source is spiritual energy. It is composed of ideas, and man can turn on its current by making mental contact with it. We can have fullness of life by realizing that we live in a sea of abundant, omnipresent, eternal life, and by refusing to allow any thought to come in that stops the consciousness of the universal life flow.

Question Helps

1. "Life is the activity of God." Explain.
2. How is man the breath of God?
3. Why is health man's divine birthright?

4. What is the omnipresent principle of health that pervades all things?
5. What is the true purpose of healing agencies?
6. How does man contact the source of healing?

Personal Notes

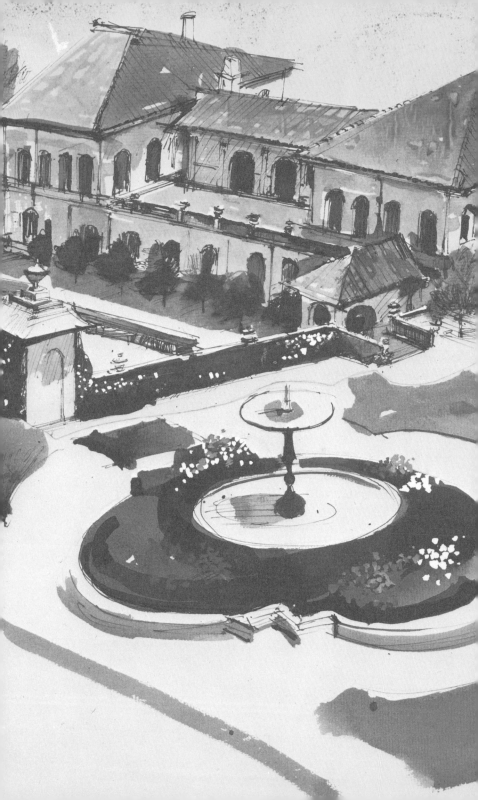

The Great Healer

Jesus revealed the divine pattern of the body as a gift from the Father, a perfect glorified creation, eternal in Mind. To Him the physical body was never the real one, because He saw beyond it to the permanent, spiritual idea existent in the infinite consciousness. If He had not so recognized it, He could never have demonstrated His power over it by overcoming death. In the Resurrection He fulfilled the divine likeness of man as conceived by the Father.

The word *holy* is from the same root as the word *heal.* Holiness and health in their root significance are the same and are a state of wholeness. In the system of Christ, holiness and health are joined. The one is the internal spiritual state; the other is the result, the outpicturing of the Christ ideas in thought, word, and act. The record of Jesus' resurrection states clearly that He assumed His natural body at will, the natural body being that which was recognized by His friends. For them, He must still bear the image of the earthly, because they could not yet discern His image of the heavenly. Christianity indicates to us not that spiritual man is without a body, but that his body is not circumscribed by limitations superimposed by self-consciousness. It teaches us that the kingdom of heaven is not entered through the gateway of death but over the top of the wall of limited mortal beliefs and that the spiritual realm is not a different place, but a different condition.

The Willingness to Live

It isn't individual healers who quicken and heal. It isn't the human desire of the individual's own heart that makes the life flow through his organism more freely. It isn't the thing that we usually think of as Christianity that brings us into the quickening, healing

13

currents of Christ life. It is the stirring in us of the same Spirit of Christ that was and is in Jesus Christ—the Spirit of God, standing forth in the individual as the expression of divine ideas from the mind of Being. It is the soul's willingness and effort actually to live, in daily thinking and acts, the Spirit of Christ, that same Spirit which made Jesus to forget Himself in doing the good and perfect will of His Father.

To believe in spiritual law, not passively but actively, is to eliminate material misconceptions and everything that is unlike God. God and His perfect creation are all there is; there is nothing else. When we understand and definitely apply spiritual principles, healing of body and affairs is not to be regarded as a supernatural feat but a natural result. It is the normal and orderly process of life in operation. Health is natural, and disease is unnatural. Jesus was the perfect expression of God-Mind. Through His spiritualized mentality, He awakened the image of the perfect pattern of the God-Mind in those who came to Him for help. By arousing their souls' energy to such an extent that the physical became immersed in healing life, He enabled the perfect man to come into manifestation. Such healing, spiritual healing, is not an attempt to gain special favor with God or to abrogate the divine or natural law. Spiritual healing is possible simply because man is a spiritual being, and health is the normal condition of man.

Reaching Out toward Life

Jesus was not concerned about the physical aspects of disease when He performed His healings. He could perform instantaneous healings because of His ability to rise to the heights of the Christ consciousness where there is no disease. He could clearly perceive man's wholeness and instantly wiped from His own and the patient's mind all that appeared as disease. He did not worry about becoming infected Himself, even when He came into contact with those suffering the effects of

14

leprosy. He did not use medical techniques as we know them today. He did not study with doctors, but rather went periodically to the wilderness, either alone or with the apostles, to commune with God and to develop divine understanding. He healed through God's power flowing through Him. He knew of the infinite energy and perfect life force contained within each man, and He simply reached out toward that life, revitalizing and energizing it, so that perfect health was instantly made manifest. Physiology teaches that the body is alive to the degree that the cells are alive, that we carry with us many dead cells. Jesus knew how to quicken with new life the cells of His own organism, and He promised that all who would follow Him would do likewise.

The Christ Presence

Jesus Christ is not merely a divine man who lived many centuries ago and whose life and works are to be considered past history. He is alive today. He is with us now. Jesus' soul radiation was so powerful that it perpetually stimulates to greater achievement and thrills with new life all who enter its sphere of influence. The Christ presence within our own souls is the Great Physician who has wisdom and power to heal and to adjust in divine order every function of our bodies. Turning within to Him, we receive that guidance, that assurance, that healing for which we long. Instead of thinking of the Lord as the personal Jesus Christ who is away in some distant heaven, we can begin to think of the Lord as our own God-given Christ Mind and of Jesus Christ as ever with us in the spiritual consciousness that He has established in the race mind so that we may be in touch with Him and build our lives according to His pattern.

Creative Healing Principles

We have thought that we were to be saved by Jesus' making personal petitions and sacrifices for us, but now we see that we are to be saved by using the creative principles that He developed in Himself and that He is ever ready to help us develop in ourselves. Recent inquiries have found His healing methods to be based on universal and spiritual laws that anyone can utilize by complying with their conditions. Thus we see that when Jesus said, "He who hears my word . . . has eternal life," He meant that we should realize the life-giving properties of the words of God as He realized them, that we should have no consciousness of death. To attain this realization of the word of life we must create currents of energy in our bodies as Jesus did in His. Although many persons doubt at this time the mind's ability to know consciously how relative substance is formed, there are those who have made contact with the thought processes and can apply them in transforming the cells and tissues of their own bodies. There are in the world today men and women who have followed the teaching of Jesus and have developed in their bodies a superenergy that permeates the physical structure. Spirit reveals that spiritual thinking breaks open the physical cells and atoms and releases the imprisoned life that originated in Divine Mind. Jesus carried this process so far that His whole body was transformed and became a conscious part of the Father-life and intelligence. The body and the blood of Jesus were purified, and each cell was energized with original spiritual substance and life until all materiality was purged away and only the pure essence remained. This essence of life and substance was sown as seed in the race consciousness, and whoever through faith in Christ draws to himself one of these germs becomes inoculated with Jesus Christ quality, and not only his mind but also his body is renewed.

God loves spiritual man, and that love is expressed according to exact law. It is not emotional or variable, nor is there any taint of partiality in it. We are primarily spiritual beings, expressions of God's perfection. When we think and act in the consciousness of perfection and love, we cannot help being open to the influx of God's love and to the fulfillment of His divine purpose. Matter *per se* does not exist; it seems to exist because of our present limitation of vision—the impermanent movement of thought not based on spiritual discernment of the eternal verities. We are not what we appear to be. We are spirit, of the Spirit of God, intrinsically perfect in God's perfectness. The resurrection of Jesus from the tomb proved conclusively that man is not a material being, subject to the laws of matter. Sense testimony gives us the conviction that man is mortal and material, under bondage to physical laws, but the Resurrection disproved this most fixed of mortal beliefs.

Jesus saw only the perfection of the spiritual body; He knew that the material body is formed out of the idea of perfection and that it does not exist in its own right. With the correct conception of the true body, the material body becomes perfect. Because the flesh registers the thought, Jesus saved His body from corruption and carried it into the heavenly zone. By following His method, we can do what He did.

In the infancy of man's spiritual development, he may find various physical and mental healing means helpful and important to him, but the ultimate goal is, "You, therefore, must be perfect, as your heavenly Father is perfect." The ultimate is not even to have faith enough to pray for healing through spiritual means. The ultimate is to *be* whole and to live in that wholeness continuously. Healing is opened to us through the Christ of our own being. To be healed through a practitioner is to be healed in proportion to the practicioner's measure of understanding. To be healed through Christ is to be healed in the measure of the Christ understanding: "I and the Father are one." We are never separated from the Great Physician, and no condition is "hopeless." All can be made whole and perfect—not just patched up, but completely and eternally whole.

Question Helps

1. Explain how holiness and healing are related.
2. When does healing of the body and affairs become a natural result instead of a supernatural feat?
3. How is Jesus Christ alive today?
4. How can individuals utilize Christ's healing principles?
5. "Man is primarily a spiritual being—the expression of God's perfection." Explain.
6. What is man's ultimate goal in spiritual healing?

Personal Notes

God's Greatest Gift

The most inclusive name for Being is Jehovah God. Jehovah represents the individual I AM and God, the universal principle. When man thinks or says "I am," he is potentially giving freedom to the seed idea that contains in its spiritual capacity all of Being. The natural man in his narrowed mental comprehension barely touches the seed ideas that expand in the Christ man to infinite power. The more we dwell upon and expand our I AM the greater looms its originating capacity in us. Jesus realized that the I AM preceded all manifestation, however great, and was capable of infinite expression.

The Scriptures plainly teach that men may become gods. When man realizes that "death and life are in the power of the tongue" and begins to use his "I am" statements wisely, he has the key that unlocks the secret chambers of existence in heaven and Earth. As the mind incorporates ideas from the one divine Source, it enlarges its brain area and gives increased mental and spiritual ability to the whole man. Jesus Christ has shown us the way that man will be transformed from flesh and blood into the glory of radiant mind.

Releasing Spiritual Energy

The energy available in our minds is unlimited; we need only learn to conserve and properly utilize it. When we learn to do this, we will effortlessly restore the body and illumine the mind. With every thought there is a radiation of energy. If a person is untrained in thinking and lets his mind express all kinds of thoughts without control, he not only uses up his thought stuff but also fails to accomplish any helpful result. The metaphysician handles omnipresent Spirit life and substance very much as the electrician handles electricity. Energy is locked up in all life and substance, and its release enables the metaphysician to utilize it in demonstrating health. When we learn to affirm "I am," with our thoughts centered on Spirit, we quicken the life flow in the body and awaken the sleepy cells. Such affirmations clear up congested areas of the organism and restore the circulation to its normal state, health. When man directs the power of exalted ideas into his body, he exalts the cells and releases their innate spiritual energy. Ability to pick up the life current and through it perpetually to vitalize the body is based on the right relation of ideas, thoughts, and words. These mental impulses start currents of energy that form and also stimulate molecules and cells already formed, producing life, strength, and animation where inertia and impotence were the dominant appearance. This was and is the healing method of Jesus. By the word which controls manifestation, Jesus Christ healed and still heals physical ills. This healing is His temporal ministry. By opening to us the avenue of return to God, Jesus Christ heals us spiritually. This healing is His eternal ministry. After the spiritual healing is accomplished, there will be no cry for physical healing. The soul being restored to wholeness, the body will be restored to soundness.

Abundant Life

Life is God's gift. The outer life is but the overflowing of the inner life, and this inner life is fed from the fountain of life through Christ at the center of our being. God gives His own life freely to all who can receive it. God's gifts are to all alike, but we have to learn how to receive freely that which He gives, how to open ourselves to the inflow of divine life through the Christ at the center of our being, exactly as we would open ourselves to the warm rays of the sun.

Jesus came that we might have life and that we might "have it abundantly." He came to show us our true relation to the source of all life, and to teach us how to draw consciously on God for more abundant life as we need it. This abundant life is always present. When we recognize it and open our consciousness to it, it comes flowing into mind and body with its mighty quickening, healing power, and they are renewed and transformed. The greatest gift of God is life itself, and we stir up this life by affirming life, by refusing to let ourselves fall into negative, defeating attitudes of mind or routines of living. The more energy we use, the more energy is released in us. We have all had times when we felt alive with energy, when our work seemed to flow through our hands, when it seemed that we accomplished things in half the ordinary time, and still felt fresh, untired, alive. This is our natural state, and through a greater understanding of our own being, we can make this feeling of unfailing energy a permanent aspect of our lives.

The life force in the body is an invisible, constuctive, intelligent force that even science cannot explain. This silent, invisible force builds the body, keeps it in repair, and cleverly operates it by processes that the personality dwelling in it does not need to understand or direct. Thus each individual is provided with a body the functions and growth of which are controlled by an intelligence that is beyond his comprehension. However, each individual is able to disrupt the perfect functioning of the life forces in his body by thinking thoughts and doing things that are not in accord with the intelligent force that directs the automatic functions and growth. This intelligent force is also known as God, and God is principle—definite, exact, and unchangeable rules of action. God is mind. Mind evolves ideas. These ideas are evolved in an orderly way. The laws of mind are just as exact and undeviating as the laws of mathematics or music. To recognize this is the starting point in finding God. As soon as man comes to this realization, he can begin to follow and uphold these laws rather than work against them, and thereby demonstrate perfect health. Each man uses the life principle according to his consciousness, inviting either health or sickness. The individual who is "strong in the Lord" (or law) of his being will not succumb to the attacks of adverse microorganisms as will the person whose innate energies and resources are weakened by fear, hatred, jealousy, and other destructive factors in his experience.

Speaking and Thinking Life

Men are to be alive: not merely to exist in a half-dead way for a few years and then go out with a sputter like a candle. Jesus Christ's men are to be electric lights that glow and gleam with perpetual current from the one omnipresent energy. The connection with that current is to be made through the mind by setting up sympathetic energies. Perfect health is natural, innate, and can be spoken into expression. Our ills are the result of our failure to adjust our minds to Divine Mind. When the right state of mind is established, man is restored to his primal and natural wholeness. This is wholly a mental process, and so all conditions of man are the result of his thinking. "As he thinketh in his heart, so is he." All conscious taking or receiving from God is a mental process. The human mind believes itself, in the matter of life, cut off from God, a separate being, something apart from God. This belief is not correct. The wire of communication between the Creator and His creations is never cut, the channel of inflowing divine life never closed.

Do you need healing? God is in the midst of you as life. God's life is the only life, and this is the life that fills your body, this is the life that flows in and through every part of you. There is no condition that is beyond God's power to heal; there is no disease that is resistant to God's healing life.

The Life of the Body

The body, which is made up of the action of thoughts of life, love, substance, power, and intelligence, is never

22

old. The very substance that gives the body its form and that nourishes and sustains it is ever new and responsive to the thoughts of life that are impressed upon it. The body is entirely renewed in less than a year, and one can renew and rebuild it and change its appearance by changing one's thoughts and living habits. Man was created as both a physical and a spiritual being and was given dominion and power to create his body according to his mental images. "God is Spirit." "Do you not know that your body is a temple of the Holy Spirit within you, which you have from God?" If God is Spirit and dwells in man's body, that body must have within it certain spiritual principles. Here modern science comes to the rescue of primitive Christianity, telling us that the atoms that compose the cells of our bodies have within them electrical units that, released, can change the whole character of the organism. Our physical bodies are carried in our minds as thought, and the body obediently reflects every mental attitude. When in the course of our evolution we discern that an all-wise Creator must have designed perfection for all His creation and we begin to affirm that perfection, then the transformation from the natural to the spiritual body begins and perfect wholeness is manifested.

The religions of every race have taught this perfection of the body but have usually assumed that it was to be given to God's elect in some heavenly place after death. They have not thought it possible that the body of flesh with its many apparent defects could be transformed into an ideal body. In consequence man has put the stamp of inferiority upon his body, and through the creative power of thought he has built into the race mind a consciousness of corruptible flesh instead of the inherent incorruptible substance of God-Mind. That the body of flesh has within it life elements that can be released and incorporated into a much finer body has always been beyond the comprehension of the sense mind, and it required a physical demonstration to con-

23

vince men that it could be done. Jesus made that demonstration.

People have not made much progress through the centuries, because they have concentrated on imitating Jesus Christ's acts instead of imitating His words and thoughts. They did not realize that outer manifestation is the result, not the cause. It is to this inner realm of thought that we must look for the transforming power of man and of the world. "Be transformed by the renewal of your mind." Mind is the link between God and man, and it is through correct understanding and use of the power of thought that man can manifest perfection in his body and in his world. Man must strive to develop his spiritual self and not be too concerned with the personal man. Imperfections in the body can occur only when the human mind is not fully cooperating with the perfect spiritual man. The mind of the individual influences the state of health in the body. Disorder in any part of the body indicates a wrong attitude in the mind. Man and the universe are founded on mind and all changes for good or ill are changes of mind. The present material universe is a product of men's thought, based on the idea of perfect order in God-Mind. It can be returned to a state of perfection if man will quit identifying with materiality and know himself as Spirit.

The body is the individual's specific interpretation of himself. The body is a record of his thoughts and man can express (appear as) any sort of body that he can conceive. We must cast off old misconceptions that our body is flesh, finite, corruptible—for it is Spirit. There is no separation between the spiritual man and the personal, except that which man himself creates through his thought. If we make a separation in our consciousness, we shall have something that we do not know how to deal with. The body is God's temple, used to bring His Spirit to work on Earth, and man has no right to think anything but perfection about it.

The body is like a child: it needs constant prompting and training and discipline and praise and appreciation. The body is perfectly equipped to do the work of Spirit on Earth; you need only allow Spirit to work through you. Look at your chest: it breathes in the very breath of God's life; God is flowing through it to supply all your needs. Look at your legs and feet: God has created them to enable you to walk on the earth, to move about freely and to do that which gives you practical knowledge of life on this plane. Your head is wonderfully poised, so that you may look about and see the beauty and light of God manifested in His creation everywhere. The body is equipped to maintain itself in health, to cure itself of disease, and to remain youthful by successfully coping with the factors that bring about what we call "old age." Many doctors have long held that all sickness in human experience is caused by a congestion or strangulation of the flow of the life forces through the body. Sickness, weakness, and deterioration originate with the strangulating effects of fear, worry, and tension. Studies in the medical field are pointing clearly and inescapably to the validity of health through spiritual means, through a conscious awareness of the stress-free spiritual dimension of life.

Realization of Perfection

If all the prayers and mind efforts of literary geniuses were inquired into, it would be found that they were wrought by heroic mental effort. So it is with healing. The realization of perfection takes root in the soul and may come forth in a flash as perfect health. The free flow of God's life through us becomes hindered in its expression if our thoughts and acts imply a belief in a limited number of years, in a hoarding of strength or substance or supply. God in the midst of us is a great steady stream of renewing, cleansing, vitalizing life, and we can have the use of this life if we will open up the channels of its flowing and draw from this source.

God does not afflict us with disease or other forms of negation even to test or try the powers with which He has endowed us. He has, however, given us the power of choice, and we may by thought, emotion, word, or act choose some form of negation. The power of Spirit is greater than human thought, emotion, word, or action and is powerful to erase the results of mistaken human direction. It is up to us not to ascribe more power to our human mistakes than we do to the power of God and not to let mistakes rule our lives.

In the dawn of creation, God established the law, everything bringing forth after its own kind. This law is still at work in every aspect of the earth today. "Whatever a man sows, that he will also reap." This law, like the word of God, is a two-edged sword. Granting that the law is inexorable, we watch for its action in our world of body, mind, and spirit. We see a relationship between states of mind and emotion and bodily conditions. The damaging effect upon the body of long-held destructive thoughts and emotions, long suspected by the metaphysically minded, now has the acceptance of medical science.

Just as the law is seen to operate in negative ways, it is tremendously powerful to act in positive ways. The same law by which we may have worked ourselves into a quagmire of trouble can surely bring us safely, triumphantly, out of it. Man must put himself in harmony with the law, then all difficulties disappear; he must replace error with Truth.

Eternal and Perfect Life

Jesus showed by His life and teachings that it is the will of God for men to be well. A clear understanding of this is necessary if one wants to demonstrate health. Where there is a belief that God wills sickness and suffering, His love and power are shut out of consciousness. Spiritual healing depends on faith, and there cannot be faith while the mind is holding thoughts directly opposed to the possibility of healing. It is therefore very necessary to dwell much on the love and power of God so that a steady, unwavering faith may be established. God is all-good; He can be nothing of disease, hate, or broken relationships. Those are outside Him. His will for us in only good. We need only follow our own inner Christ nature in order to get in harmony with all good and manifest perfection in our bodies.

We must think life, talk life, and see ourselves filled with the fullness of life. When we are not manifesting life as we desire, it is because our thoughts and our conversations are not in accord with the life idea. Every time we think life, speak life, rejoice in life, we are setting free and bringing into expression in ourselves more and more of the life idea. In this way we enter into the same consciousness of abundant, enduring, unfailing, eternal life that Jesus had, and we can readily understand His proclamation that those who believe in the indwelling Christ life will never die.

Question Helps

1. How does affirming "I am" quicken the life flow in the body?
2. What is God's greatest gift to man? Why?
3. How can man make the feeling of unfailing energy a permanent aspect of life?
4. Define "life force."
5. How does the mind of the individual influence the state of health in the body?
6. Can individuals enter into the same consciousness of abundant, eternal life that Jesus Christ had? Explain.

Personal Notes

The Power of the Word

Spiritual psychology proves that the name of a great character carries his mind potency and that wherever his name is repeated silently or audibly, his attributes become manifest. Jesus demonstrated that He understood the healing power stored up in the body, which He said is released through faith. "Your faith has made you well." Each of us can call on Jesus' name to release stored healing life in our own body. Any declaration which man makes in which the name *Jesus Christ* is used reverently will contact the spiritual ether where the Christ I AM exists and will open the mind and body to the inflow of spiritual healing energy. The name *Jesus Christ* holds all power within it. The words *Jesus Christ,* with all their original meaning behind them and embodied in them, produce spiritual vibrations of infinite fineness and power.

Speaking with Spiritual Authority

When a person is given authority to speak or to act in the name of a king or of a chief executive, his speaking or acting carries with it the full power vested in the ruler together with that of the entire government behind him. When we speak with full authority, using the name of Jesus Christ—the anointed Son of God, the Savior to whom has been given "all authority in heaven and on Earth"—we set in motion a mighty though invisible force to accomplish that whereto our words are sent. Thus, when we pray in the name and through the power of Jesus Christ, Christ's Spirit is invoked and His power flows through us, so it is not our power alone that is at work, but all power for good that exists. The mental harmony of Jesus not only radiates throughout the Earth but reaches into the heavens, where it taps the glory of God. When we pray in the name of the Lord Jesus Christ or decree His presence and power in our spiritual work, we effect a reunion with His supermind and its tremendous ramifications in heaven and Earth, and our own meager spiritual abilities are augmented a thousandfold.

For two thousand years those who have had faith in Jesus and proclaimed their faith in His name have had proof that He is present as a dynamic life-giving force. Men and women with no previous healing power have suddenly become healers of marvelous ability. They do not claim to understand how the healing is done. They know only that through the exercise of faith and their word, the spiritual quality in them is fused into unity with the power of Christ and the work is marvelously accomplished.

That the name of Jesus Christ is a real, practical, wonder-working, result-producing power there is no doubt. Many instances of spiritual healings are related in the New Testament. In the Acts of the Apostles we find that, following the death and resurrection of Jesus, Peter and John one day instantly healed "a man lame from birth . . . whom they laid daily at that gate of the temple which is called Beautiful to ask alms." This healing was done through Peter by the spoken word: "In the name of Jesus Christ of Nazareth, walk." The story continues by relating that "immediately his feet and ankles were made strong. And leaping up he stood and walked and entered the temple with them, walking and leaping and praising God. And all the people saw him walking and praising God, and recognized him as the one who sat for alms at the Beautiful Gate of the temple; and they were filled with wonder and amazement at what had happened to him. . . . And when Peter saw it he addressed the people, 'Men of Israel, why do you wonder at this, or why do you stare at us, as though by our own power or piety we had made him walk? The God of Abraham and of Isaac and of Jacob, the God of our fathers, glorified his servant Jesus. . . . And his name, by faith in his name, has made this man strong.' "

Healing of Mind and Body

The Master emphasized the true authority of His teaching by definite physical effects. He was not satisfied to minister to the spirit and ignore the flesh. His ministrations were joint healings of mind and body. Few people realize that health includes more than just the flesh body. In fact it is unknown to most people that the body is but a result of mental and spiritual activity, and that that person is healthiest who best maintains a true balance among spirit, mind, and body. Not many think of health as an expression of divine intelligence, a radiation of infinite energy, a liberation of God's activity. To Jesus, spirit and body were inseparable and indistinguishable. He did not quibble over doctrine, but gave physical demonstration when it was demanded. His "Rise, take up your bed and go home" was the material demonstration of the real healing that had already been accomplished. If the primitive minds of the people more readily understood a physical result than a spiritual cause, Jesus was willing to let them have it their way.

To keep the word of Jesus means to awaken to the inner life and the world of Spirit; hence man must take up spiritual ways. We must not keep merely the letter of the word, but keep its spirit by getting right where Jesus Christ was in relation to the world and grasping His words with our minds. One cannot get Spirit and life out of matter and death. Unless one perceives that there is something more in the doctrine of Jesus than keeping up a worldly moral standard as preparation for salvation after death, he will fall short of being a real Christian.

Words of Truth

In about twenty places in the New Testament, Jesus is recorded as saying in substance, "Follow me." It is evident that He meant for us to follow His example of

31

being receptive to God's wisdom, peace, power, and health. In the instance of the man at the pool of Bethesda, a man who had been ill for thirty-eight years, Jesus said to him, "Do you want to be healed?" The man replied that no man would help him, and Jesus said, "Rise, take up your pallet, and walk." The man was made whole, and took up his pallet and walked. This healing represents the power of the Christ (typified by Jesus) to restore the equilibrium of the organism through the activity of spiritual ideas in consciousness, independently of the healing methods utilized by the sense man. The true spiritual healing method employs the word of authority, as spoken by Jesus, which must be set into activity. Through the power of the word the "infirmity" gives place to perfect equalization and strength.

All words of Truth are alive with an invisible energy that has power to work miracles. Truth is mighty to accomplish results, but in order to do so it must be spoken into activity. Life, Truth, Christ are one. The words of Truth that you and I speak in the name and Spirit of the Master become His words, full of life and health. Such words set into motion the invisible energy that accomplishes results, and nothing is accomplished when it is quiescent.

Speaking definite, positive words of assurance to oneself or to another has marvelous power to lift and transform, power to fill the body with a consciousness of the real living presence of God. This is God's way of delivering us out of our troubles. He comforts us and gives us newness of life through our speaking words of Truth to ourselves and to Him. Such words have power to free the channel between our own center of life and the fountain of all life—a channel that may have become clogged by our selfishness or ignorance—so that a great, surging influx of new life can take place. Every instant that our hearts are uplifted in the spirit of gratitude, which is aroused by our speaking words of thanks for benefits already received, this mighty energy that is the Spirit of the living God is working to change, restore, and heal the very trouble that seems about to destroy us.

Words of Truth from a zealous man possess dynamic power to heal and bless because the spiritual man enters into them. When the zone of Spirit, from which healing words emanate, is unobstructed, they feed the souls of men and are creative as well as re-creative. The word of Truth has life in it; it has power to restore and make whole; it cannot perish or grow less with the changes that come with the passing years. The more spiritual the individual who gives forth the words, the more enduring they are; the more powerfully the words move men, the more surely they awaken them to their divine nature.

Jesus said, "Keep my word," meaning to resolve it in the mind, to go over it in all its aspects, to believe in it as a truth, and to treasure it as a saving, healing balm in time of need. Words have powers to cast out demons and to heal the sick.

Whatever the various theories of Jesus' remarkable healing power may be, none disputes one point: He used words as the vehicle of the healing potency. He had a certain assurance, an inner conviction, that He was speaking the truth when He said, "You are well!" and the result of His understanding carried conviction to the mind of the patient and opened the way for the healing.

Words are quickened by those who speak them; they pick up and carry the ideas of the speaker, weak or strong, ignorant or wise, good or ill. Thus words descriptive of deity have been personalized in the thought stuff of the race, and those who invoke them in prayer and meditation are given a spiritual impetus far beyond what they would receive from common words. Next to Spirit, the word of Spirit is the most powerful thing in existence. "The world was created by the word of God." We read in Genesis that "God said . . ." and it came to pass. God said, "Let us make man in our own image, after our likeness." Thus we see that man is the incarnate word of God, and that our own words bring forth whatever we put into them.

The Only Creative Power

If one would be healed, let him study the healing words of Jesus. Let him take these words into his consciousness. Doing this, he will at once receive ameliorating aid. If he persists in the study, he will prosper in his search for God, and ultimately will be thoroughly, eternally healed. Jesus did not copyright His words or forbid anyone else to use them. He importuned you and me to keep them as He kept them—right in His heart—to realize that this is no idle repetition of words but the setting up of a living fire in the soul.

Jesus' words are varied, but all are food for the minds of men. None of them is too difficult for us or too far from our present power of realization.

Our words bring about in our lives and affairs whatever we put into them. Through the law of expression and form, words of weakness change to weakness the character of everything that receives them. Talking about nervousness and weakness will produce corresponding conditions in the body; on the other hand, sending forth the word of strength and affirming power will bring about strength and poise. Nerves carry thought-messages to every part of the body, where the thoughts manifest the word "spoken" to them. Words set up a particular vibration with their intonation, and we can affect our own or others' life vibrations by our manner of addressing them. By telling the little child that he looks sick and tired, the mother produces these conditions in the child's mind and body. If the mother addresses words of health, life, and strength to the child, these will set his bodily functions into activity and they will express the harmony of the dominant thought. Every word brings forth after its kind.

The perfect Word of God is spiritual man. It is through spiritual man that all things are brought into manifestation. As an imitator of Divine Mind, man has the power to form and make manifest whatsoever he idealizes, but unless his thought is unified with Divine Mind and guided in its operations by infinite wisdom, his thought forms are perishable.

Mind is the one and only creative power. Following the creative law in its operation from the formless to the formed, we can see how an idea fundamental in Divine Mind is grasped by man's ego, how it takes form in his thought, and how it is expressed through his spoken word. If in each step of this process he conformed to the divine creative law, man's word would make things instantly, as Jesus made the increase of the loaves and fishes. But since he has lost, in a measure, knowledge of the steps in this creative process from the within to the without, there are many breaks and abnormal conditions, with more failures than success in the products. But every word, thought or uttered, has some effect.

If the reasonable premise that God is the omnipresent God is well grounded in you, you cannot speak anything but healing and uplifting words. If you believe that both good and evil conditions can be brought forth from Divine Mind, however, then your healing will be mixed. The stream is pure; you limit it in its expression by your error thinking.

Anyone can speak true words and thus be the agent of God. The little child may do it; the ignorant disciple may do it. The power does not inhere in the individual. The living Word of God is spiritual principle. It is omnipresent, like the air we breathe, and anyone may apply it. Its premise is that God is good and that His offspring is like Him. You have only to recognize this premise in all that you think and do, and then speak it forth to get the results promised.

Question Helps

1. How does calling on the name of Jesus Christ release stored healing life?
2. What does it mean to keep the word of Jesus?
3. Explain how words are quickened.
4. Why is spiritual man the perfect Word of God?
5. "Mind is the one and only creative power." Explain.

Personal Notes

Man's Creative Thought

Man is not a flesh body resulting from a material conception, but a creation of Spirit, a manifestation of his own individual thought. "As he thinketh in his heart, so is he." He cannot change his state of mind without automatically causing a corresponding change in his body. Man's body is an orderly record of his self-discoveries, an outpicturing of his interpretation of the functions and powers that are originally his by divine right. It is a cosmic law that thoughts become things. It is the creative essence of all phenomena. Whether we believe it or not and whether our thoughts are adverse or harmonious, they objectify themselves and create the character of our surroundings. An impression received and recorded by the consciousness of the individual enters the subconsciousness as a belief, and from that moment, whether it is true or false, it proceeds to exercise dominion. We see, then, how necessary it is to know the truth and to train the consciousness to allow no unchallenged thought to enter its realm.

The Mental Model of the Body

The body of man is an effect, a manifestation of all that he has believed about it, an externalization of the idea that his soul has formed of itself. It is thus a continuous creation of the mind, just as the soul is a perpetual creation of God. It would be foolish to deny the existence of the body, but we know that it has no independent existence. It continually derives its being from the mind. As a body it has neither life nor power. Without the consciousness that it expresses, it could do nothing. But on the other hand, neither could the consciousness become expression without an organism. Mind and body must work together in fulfilling the divine purpose—the manifestation of infinite goodness.

So much for the original idea or divine plan. The human race has worked it out very differently. It has bound and limited its consciousness with error. It has believed in a material, corruptible, destructible flesh body, something that suffers pain and injury and dies. It has bequeathed this inheritance to every man. In attempting to free himself from what he feels to be a false conception, man has gone to the opposite extreme and denied his body, constantly thinking of himself as Spirit only, and this belief in separateness manifests itself as such unless it is given the protection of Truth principles.

The body is an individual record of thought and identifies each person's interpretation of what he has "learned" through his physical senses. If he has believed in their report of the subconscious impression of race thought, his body will publish the fact. The truth found in Christianity destroys this belief concerning the body and discerns the real or "Lord's body" that is man's perfect identity in God.

In the infinite plan there was never such a creation as a body of flesh; there was no such manifestation as that which so tormented Paul with its contrary way of always doing as he "would not" and not doing as he "would." Man is continually perfect in Divine Mind. But our sense consciousness continues to read the thoughts of those about us as expressed in their bodies and, by the same sign, to recognize the change of thought as it manifests itself in altered bodies and different conditions. Concealment is impossible. There is nothing hidden away in a man's thought that is not revealed in his body and his life. He furnishes the mental model that his body images forth, and the bodily impression is a true representation of what he has chosen to think in his heart.

Man's Mental Resurrection

All nature renews itself periodically. Man may use his relationship with nature to rejuvenate himself. As

God creates the universe by divine ideas, so man may re-create his body by his governing thought. Every new and higher conception he forms will tend to an outward bodily expression. This transformation must be wrought by the individual himself and comes through the annihilation of ignorance and error rather than as the result of physical death. It may be accounted a mental resurrection, and it is man's privilege to rise from the grave of false thinking. The mind works from any model we furnish it. If we hold steadfastly before it the divine idea and believe in its realization, it will re-create the body in accordance with its mental pattern. The body is healed only as the thought is healed. There is but one Mind, and the health of man's body, being in the Mind, can never be impaired or lost. When the concept of this spiritual body is revealed to man, healing becomes the most normal thing in the world. It is impossible for the body to manifest pain or disease if the thought which miscreated it is destroyed.

Unlimited Power

There is a universal thought substance in which thought builds whatever man wills. Man has unlimited power through thought, and he can give his power to things or withhold it. His whole character is determined by the thoughts for which he allows a place in his mind. A strong man or a weak man is what he is because of repeated thoughts of strengh or weakness. Everything we see around us is the creation of Mind, molded by thought. All the conditions of this world have been constructed by the people who inhabit the world, and each individual is a builder of and personally responsible for his immediate environment. Jesus Christ set out to establish the kingdom of heaven on Earth by awakening men to this fundamental truth of being. He taught the power of mind, thoughts, words. He cast out demons (error thoughts) and healed the sick with a word.

We are mind. Our consciousness is formed of thoughts. Thoughts form barriers about the thinker, and when accepted as true they are impregnable to other thoughts. So we are compassed about with thought barriers, the result of our heredity, our education, our own thinking. Likewise our degree of health is determined by our thoughts, past and present. These thoughts may be true or false, depending on our understanding and use of divine law. We lose our health when we cease to follow universal law, either by omission or commission. To be continuously healthy we must draw on the one and only source of life, God.

God does not form things. God calls from the depths of His own Being the ideas that are already there, and they move forth and clothe themselves with the habiliments of time and circumstance in man's consciousness. Man is that which he wills himself to be. He is not a puppet to be controlled by an omnipotent outer power, but a living, breathing, cooperating being who knows the thoughts and desires of Divine Mind and cooperates with it in bringing about the ends of a perfect and healthy creation. Within man there is a capacity for knowing God consciously and for communing with Him. Man was not created as an inferior being, but in fellowship with his Creator. He therefore creates by means of his word and his thought, just as God creates. Each spoken work has power to cause to manifest that which it decrees, especially those words spoken with spiritual consciousness. Every act and every condition has its origin in the mind. Thoughts, whether negative or positive, are seeds that, when dropped or planted in the subconscious mind, germinate, grow, and bring forth their fruit in due season. The mind reacts to ideas, and ideas are made visible in words. Hence the holding of right words in the mind will set the mind going at a rate proportioned to the dynamic power of the idea back of the words. A word with a lazy idea back of it will not stimulate the mind or heal the body. The words must represent swift, strong spiritual ideas if they are to infuse the mind with energy. These are the kinds of words that Jesus reveled in. He delighted in making great and mighty claims for His God, for Himself, for His works, and for all men. With these powerful words, He healed the sick and raised the dead.

Seeking to Express Perfection

The way to healing is first to reeducate the mind and to establish the presence of Truth in all the faculties. Then one must see the reality of the body and its functions and stamp every part with the perfect pattern which is the outpicturing of Christ ideas in individual consciousness. One must study his living habits and make them conform to the truth that good only is real, abiding, and truly active. When a person holds the thought that his body is pure, alive, and perfect in every part and uses this mental pattern to direct him in his thoughts and living habits, no disease can touch him. By reeducating his mind and reshaping his mental patterns, he causes the outpicturing in his body to become perfect.

The individual must do it himself, but he can know that God is working through him constantly. When our own consciousness corresponds to God's perfect idea of us, we will express that perfection in every aspect of our physical being. The one who is truly seeking that which is of God is expressing the good and the true in thought. He does not think adverse thoughts or believe in impurity of any sort in the self or in others.

Concentration on the Perfect Pattern

All the senses work in the realm of mind, but all have their physical side and use. We use what they tell us in our thought world. That which we think of ourselves, of others, or of the creation in general, we build up the belief in and begin to register in our own souls and bodies. Our eyes begin to visualize that which we habitually see mentally, and the cell structures of the organs

41

themselves are affected and built according to the vibrations set up by the thoughts. This is true of the other senses and their organs. Our negative thoughts and emotions act upon the parts of the body that have to do with phases of life that they touch.

We must see the life of God in our flesh. Any form of denial of God-life and intelligence or of the physical organism, any thought of the flesh other than as of God's pure substance, congests and irritates the body. This is double-mindedness, a believing in evil as well as good. To look about one and see evil and imperfection is sinful. That which we mentally stamp a thing is registered in our own flesh. Man must conserve and regulate this thought energy in order to develop right thinking. Right thinking is using the mind to bring about right ends idealized by the thinker. Man controls the demonstration of health in his body according to his control and conservation of thought force. The perfect body exists as an ideal body in us all. By mentally concentrating on this perfect body (the Christ-body) and focusing all our powers on it as the vital life of the physical, a transformation will begin that will finally raise the physical to divine stature.

We cannot be healed by thinking about sickness, nor can we be prospered by thinking about lack. Every time we dwell on a thought of limitation about our lives—a thought of disease or age or death—we cause a restriction in the flow of life. The strange thing is that often a person may be praying for healing and all the while restricting the flow of life and wholeness because he is fearfully dwelling on the condition he is afraid of and does not want. If we feel frustrated while praying for a condition that does not seem to improve, our frustration may actually cause the condition to worsen. We nourish negative conditions by dwelling upon them, mourning them, and wishing they were not there. Rather, direct your thought *away from* negative conditions. Do not think of them at all, and they will disappear. We may nourish a good thing by thinking how good it is—a beautiful face, a beautiful form, whatever it may be that is good; but if we take the negative side, we shall then get results also. We shall get just what we think about. Our minds draw upon the vital forces, and according to psychological laws we alter our tissues. The mind acts on the body through the nerves, and either we tear down our bodies or we build them up.

Disease

Thoughts of a certain type produce physical conditions which we know as disease. They bring about a mental chemistry that produces a change of the chemical contents in the body, thereby producing abnormal or pathological conditions. In some instances thought produces a congestion of blood in one part, thereby robbing another part of the body of the blood supply it should have. Even the simplest thought of self-consciousness will cause a person's face to flush with an abnormal supply of blood. We also have the instance of the individual who through a thought of fear causes his face to blanch as the blood supply is kept from circulating through blood vessels in the face. What if this uneven circulation were kept up for a period of time? Can we doubt that thought can instantly choke off an organ's blood supply and its nutrition, or can overfeed it?

Fear keeps the stomach from properly receiving and handling foods that are eaten and causes a poison in the system which may prevent some part of the body from getting its share of nourishing food elements. Fear hinders circulation so that waste materials are not properly eliminated. Fear causes a gnawing hunger which makes the child or grown-up eat fitfully— sometimes craving things not needed, sometimes refusing beneficial foods.

We must replace error thoughts in the subconscious, such as fear and worry, with Truth statements. Our

43

body temples are the fruit of our minds. The truths that we hold in mind redeem and heal our flesh. In Spirit and in Truth we are now and always every whit whole. By getting false thoughts out of the way, by keeping the image and likeness of wholeness ever before our mind's eye, and by trying to *feel* that we are healed, health becomes irresistible and it is bound to manifest.

Affirm Divine Order

Order must be established in all areas of life. The first step is to watch our thoughts and words. We should deny negative thoughts and express only positive words. We must cultivate right, positive thinking above all else. If we think about order and harmony, our taste in material things will change. We shall desire the purest foods, and there will be more harmony in the colors we choose to wear.

There must be order in the spiritual life as well as the material life. Accept and affirm the knowledge that there is a divine plan working in your life and affirm your oneness with Divine Mind. Know that you are the offspring of God and one with His perfect wisdom. Ask for wisdom, then affirm divine order. Put yourself in unity with Spirit, and the order of Divine Mind will begin to work in your life. Harmony will be established in all your affairs. After sowing the seeds of right thought, the plants must be tended: after using the law, we must hold to its fulfillment. This is our part, and God gives the increase. You must work in divine order and not expect the harvest before the soil has been prepared or the seed sown. You have now the fruits of previous sowings. Change your thought seeds and reap what you desire. The perfect order of the law of life is established in you through your permitting the creative ideas of life, love, substance, and intelligence to direct your thoughts and the functions of your body. The omnipresent substance of God is appropriated and impressed with perfect patterns as you keep mind and heart confident that Spirit knows how to arrange for the very best manifestations to work through you. Keep your mind open for the inflow from any source of all things needed.

Be at Peace

The mind of peace precedes bodily healing. Cast out enmity and anger and affirm the peace of Jesus Christ, and your healing will be swift and sure. Steadfast affirmations of peace will harmonize the whole body structure and open the way to attainment of healthy conditions in mind and body. One of the reasons that prayers and treatments for health are not more successful is that the mind has not been put in a receptive state by affirmations of peace. The Mind of Spirit is harmonious and peaceful, and it must have a like manner of expression in man's consciousness. When a body of water is choppy with fitful currents of air, it cannot reflect objects clearly. Neither can man reflect the steady strong glow of Omnipotence when his mind is disturbed by anxious thoughts, fearful thoughts, or angry thoughts. Be at peace and your unity with God-Mind will bring you health and happiness.

Question Helps

1. Explain how man's body is a continuous creation of his mind.
2. "The body is healed only as the thought is healed." Explain.
3. What must one do in order to be continuously healthy?
4. What is the way to healing?
5. Define "right thinking."
6. How does one establish the perfect order of the law of life?

45

Personal Notes

Contacting the Source

God has made everything good so that man can use and enjoy it. Manifest man, beginning with Adam, has been following the hard way of living by experimenting to find the difference between good and evil instead of following God's instructions to follow the easy way of absolute goodness.

Man separates himself from God's perfect creation, the kingdom of heaven, by thinking that God's creation is both good and evil. This double-mindedness causes him to worry, to fear, to be unhappy, and to indulge in many negative emotions. These emotions interfere with the harmonious working of the divine life force in his body and may cause physical disorder. The secret of healing lies in lifting up the consciousness by faith into the realm of God perfection, thus clearing the way for God's original, perfect healing to be done in the body.

The Great Physician performed His miracles of healing by bringing humanity into a consciousness of direct contact with this one and only life-stream, and by linking each lesser mind with its divine source, connecting it with its central Spirit. He did not begin with the materiality of the flesh. His diagnosis penetrated far beyond paralyzed limbs and sightless eyes. These, to Him, were but changeable, unsubstantial appearances. He worked with spiritual principle in His world of reality, the mind.

Nothing that is perishable can be real. The physical body is not man's real self, for he is continually casting it off and as constantly renewing it. The real being, the I AM, is not physical. Life is a matter of consciousness, and the body is the instrument through which the mind functions on this Earthly plane.

Thinking Life-Thoughts

Thinking is the first manifestation of the living principle in man. It is that which flows forth into the body as expression. Employed constantly in one direction, it

47

becomes a fixation or habit. Disease is the result of habitual morbid or wrong thinking. This morbidity, which Jesus termed "sin," is not necessarily a continuous thought of sickness, but can be worry, tension, or fearful thoughts. All power to conquer the causes of sickness is readily available for us to use today. Belief in the Christ in man has lost none of its vitality; it is as powerful today as it was in the time of Jesus. Jesus Himself stated that those who learned from Him and used His methods could accomplish even greater works than He Himself did: all the potential is here if only we can learn to use it.

The power of God in you is healing power. The life of God in you is eternal life. This health and this life cannot be compared to worldly standards of health and life. The world looks upon health as something fleeting, something that exists today and is changed tomorrow. The world looks upon life as something that may terminate at any second. The health and life of Christ within you are unchangeable. They endure forever.

If you lose consciousness of the life within and develop a need for healing, first turn to God within and center your thought on Him. Do not claim disease for your own or acknowledge its reality. There is no power in outside conditions; the only power is that of healing and constructive Spirit. All else is delusion, a mistaken conviction, a belief in something that is nonexistent. When the world of sense tells us that there is life, power, or substance inherent in anything outside the infinite consciousness, it misleads our judgment. All sense delusion is based on a human belief that any life or intelligence can exist independently, that is, apart from the Mind of God. Sense delusion is a failure to discern spiritual reality, and it puts its trust in a lie. It believes that we see and hear with the eyes and ears of sense, instead of those of the soul.

Through constructive thought we achieve mastery over sense delusion. To construct is to build; constructive thought is a positive, conclusive, affirmative

48

method of using the mind. It is God thought and like it, creative. It releases the potentialities of the soul; it quickens bodily functions and harmonizes discordant physical effects. No one can think positively of himself as spiritually alive, well, happy, and abundantly supplied without building in his consciousness a vitalizing effect. Reality deals with the truly existing things, which are ideas. The reality of man is the sum total of God's ideas about him. He embodies those perfect ideas, although often but faintly, through his human limitation. His physical senses are always reporting the subconscious delusions of the race, and he sees in himself and others not the real or Christ man, but what each one is thinking about himself. Jesus refused to perceive anything but reality. He took away "the sins of the world" by not seeing its mistakes or criticizing its faults.

The Perfect Word

We must understand that the Father cannot be circumscribed by any human idea of Him or of what He should do for us. We must know that there is only good and that the word of God is the only permanently healing word. So long as we believe that the Father might heal at one time and not at another, we are misjudging His nature. If there is ever any limit to the healing power of the word, it is of our own manufacture.

The healing word is not a special creation to meet an emergency. It is not a patent medicine prepared to cure specific diseases. The idea that it is a healing word at all originates in our limited notion that there is something that needs healing.

God is the supreme perfection, and all His creations are perfect. It takes cognizance of the perfect only in order to bring it into manifestation. When we realize this perfection and speak words of Truth from that plane of understanding, our word goes forth and establishes that which is. It does not heal anything—in its perfection there is nothing to heal. Its office is to behold the perfection of its Being; and as we do the works of the Father, we behold and restore that which is and always was perfect. Thus he who realizes that God is the supreme perfection and that in Him can be no imperfection and who speaks forth that realization with conviction will cause all things to arrange themselves in divine order.

Trust in God

There is a way back to the original purity of the universe, a way out of poverty, ill health, and inharmony. Jesus called it the "kingdom of the heavens" and said that "all these things" should be added to those who sought it. This implies that you do not have fully to enter this kingdom in order to have the things added, but you do have to "seek." You must turn your attention in the right direction. This is the step that everybody is commanded to take. Trust God in all things, and see the result made apparent by the mental currents that you set going all about you. Your whole life will be vitalized; the scope of your world will broaden; your mind will feel quick and alert, your body free from weakness. Your fears will be dispersed and you will have a sense of security. You will be generous and patient, and your good will be able to come to you. You will have a beneficial effect on others; they will also become happier and healthier, for anyone who comes into contact with a raised consciousness is affected favorably by it. Ideas are catching, and no man can live where true ideas of wholeness and abundance and peace are being held without becoming infected with them. Health is the divine heritage of every human being.

Unity with God through Mind

God is mind. Here we touch the connecting link between God and man. The essential being of God as principle cannot be comprehended by any of the senses or

50

faculties, but the mind of man is limitless, and through it he may come in touch with divine Principle. It is the study of mind that reveals God and with this revelation comes perfect health. Man must come consciously into the peace in mind that is common to both man and God. Your own mind does not do the healing. It is the channel through which the healing Principle works. The secret of existence will never be disclosed before man takes up and masters the science of his own mind. Man's consciousness is formed of mind and its ideas, and these determine whether he is healthy or sick. Jesus knew the power of the universe to be contained in the mind; He knew He contained all the power of the Father within Him. As the body is moved by mind, so the mind is moved by ideas, and right here in the mind we find the secret of the universe: "The Father who dwells in me does his works." The supreme realization of man is his unity with God through Mind. Jesus had this realization and proclaimed it before there was any manifestation. "I and the Father are one." "He who has seen me has seen the Father."

Think of Being as an aggregation of ideas with potential creative capacity and governed in its creative processes by unalterable laws. Mentally see those ideas projected into action in an evolving, self-conscious creature with free will—man. As man develops through the combination of those original ideas, behold his arriving at a place in his evolution where he realizes his power of self-determination and consciously begins to choose among the many activities of the universe and to combine them in his own way to form his own field of activity.

Open to the Spirit

Man is threefold being: he is spirit, soul, and body. He sets into action any of the three realms of his being by concentrating his thought on them. If he thinks only of the body, the physical senses encompass all his existence. If mind and emotion are cultivated, he adds soul

51

to his consciousness. If he rises to the Absolute and comprehends Spirit, he rounds out the God-man. The inner secrets of the universe are revealed in Spirit, and Spirit is found only by those who go about looking for it in an orderly way.

Mental discipline is needed to open the mind to Spirit. The personal consciousness is like a house with all the doors and windows barred. He who lives within may hear voices without, but the doors and windows unlock from within, and it is left to him to unfasten them. The doors and windows of the mind are solidified thoughts, and they swing loose when the right word is spoken to them. Jesus voiced a whole army of right words, and if you will take up His words and make them yours, they will open all the doors of your mind to Spirit. No one else can do this for you; you must do it yourself. Truth is not revealed by one mortal to another, but by God to each of His children who is ready to receive.

In Spirit the harmonizing, healing, adjusting activity of God coincides completely with the need. However, you must get in tune with it. There is a very real sense in which God is in constant communion with you, but you must accept the truth of this—in effect, get in communion with *Him*. You cannot hear beautiful music being broadcast unless your receiver is set at the proper frequency. There are radio waves all around you, but unless you are set to hear them, you will not.

This is the function of the affirmation: to lift your consciousness to the level of the answer. Healing is already complete in God-Mind, by the divine law of adjustment. But the solution becomes real in our experience only as we get in tune with the activity of the law. An affirmation does not make something true. It declares that which *is* true and opens the way for its manifestation. When you use prayer and affirmation, you are not appealing to an outside force. You are not praying, "O God, heal me," but rather you are knowing, with all the forces of your being, that your body is a center of life and light, that every atom and cell is filled with the substance of God's pure life.

Conscious Flow of Life's Energy

The conscious direction of the mind toward healing of the body is the most direct and natural healing agency, and one whose results become more and more powerful as regular times of meditation and prayer establish a conviction of the true nature of healing and a confidence in the innate creative forces within us all. Improvement is not attained by wishful thinking or by willpower, but by one's convictions. When man is convinced that healing is possible, that he deserves to be well, and that all the forces of his own being as well as the will of God are for him to be well, he removes roadblocks in the consciousness and clears the way.

The body is the servant of the mind, not the mind the servant of the body, and the body responds to our right mental attitudes. More than this, it responds to our right spiritual attitudes. It responds to our feeling of faith; it takes up the idea of wholeness, because this is its right and natural state. The functions of the body are performed smoothly and easily in the measure that we are willing to trust the power that is in every cell for life and wholeness. Our free and happy feeling about ourselves abets the healing flow, whereas our anxiety concerning our state of health can disturb and distress the natural working of the body.

Realizing the Image and Likeness

The real foundation of all effective healing is the understanding that God is Spirit and that man, His offspring, is His image and likeness, hence spiritual. Such a concept of God gives man a point of contact that is never absent; he is always in the presence and always has the support of the Father. God is never absent from His creations. He is the perpetual source of all good; He

53

can always be drawn upon. It is man who must learn to contact Him in every need.

It is our exalted ideas of God and our little ideas of ourselves that built the mental wall that separates us from Him. We have been taught that God is a mighty monarch with certain domineering characteristics who wills us to be sick or healthy, that He is of such majesty that man cannot conceive of Him. We must throw off these misconceptions and make our whole connection, spirit, soul, body—wholeness, all working in harmony. We have to lay hold of this concept of God as active eternal Principle, all-supplying substance, not as something that comes and goes. Supply of all good is limitless; we need only cultivate the habit of appropriating it.

Salvation through Jesus Christ is not accomplished by looking forward to freedom, but by realizing that we are now free through His freeing power. We have only to establish ourselves in real life and strength by understanding that the attributes of Being are omnipresent and that our affirmations of that Presence will cause us to realize that we do live, move, and have our being in eternal life and strength, right here, right now.

Seeing as God Sees

It is up to us to accept our God-given perfection for ourselves, to put aside past mistakes and untrue suggestions, and to fix our undivided attention upon the Creator of our inner pattern of perfection. This is the secret of success in all spiritual treatments. We must bring all our mental attitudes, the centers of our consciousness, and even our physical structures, to this high place in Divine Mind where we see as God sees. In this spiritual viewpoint we are able to name all that is within us according to the patterns of Spirit; we are able to use these soul qualities to outpicture rightly their true creative possibilities. The ebb and flow of spiritual thinking produce a fine essence of life which flows through the nerves and revitalizes our whole being.

The law of spiritual healing involves full receptivity on the part of the one under treatment. God does not do anything in us against our will. Whenever we have an experience of sickness, it is evidence that we have been letting go of our hold on the gifts of God. We have ceased eagerly to appropriate, assimilate, and make use of the life of Spirit through our thoughts, words, acts, living habits.

In seeking the way to health we are to pray for an understanding of our oneness with God and to claim it. We are to study this relationship so that we may know how to lay hold of the abundant life, intelligence, substance, and love of God, and build these into our souls and our bodies, that we may perfect our expression.

You live in God; He lives in you. The life you have been praying for is here, in you now. The healing you have been praying for is already accomplished, for you are one with God's healing power, right now.

A sufferer may pray that God manifest Himself as his health, but if the sufferer's comprehension of health is limited to the cessation of a pain, the answer to the prayer will be limited to the removal of the pain, and health will find no free avenue of manifestation in the man's life. Do not ask for healing of a particular symptom or a particular ailment; ask to manifest throughout your being the perfection that is your natural state. The way of fuller manifestation is to let God be the consciousness, let Him be the life within. Open up to His life; do not limit or block its flow.

Healing Now

Have you in your prayers for healing been inclined to think of healing as something to be accomplished in some future time; have you prayed for strength to bear your present misery and hoped for healing, sometime, somehow? Then you have been limiting God's healing

55

power in you. Allow it to manifest by affirming life in your whole being. Affirm, "I am Spirit, and Spirit cannot be sick."

Act now; *now* is the time to start your healing. Recognize that you are already healed, and begin the manifestation now. God's healing power is working through you now and always. Do not ask, "When shall I be healed?" Do not limit God's power by thinking that it cannot come now. Do not deny Him by thinking that some condition is beyond help, that some healing need is too hard for Him. All the healing life there is, is present with you and in you, right now. Do not be bound and put down by your feeling of disease. You are free to dispel any negative drawbacks or limitations. You are Spirit, free to act now.

God's man is hale, whole, hearty. We must realize this truth before it can manifest. A spiritual realization of health is the result of holding in consciousness a statement of health until the logic of the mind is satisfied and man receives the assurance that the fulfillment in the physical must follow. By realizing a healing prayer, man lays hold of the principle of health itself and the whole consciousness is illumined; principle (God) and man work out his health challenges together.

God is power; man is powerful. God is that indescribable reservoir of stored-up energy that manifests no potency whatever until set in motion through the consciousness of man, yet possesses an inexhaustible capacity that is beyond words to express. The force of its power when expressed is determined by man's method of expression. God is that power which creates and is irresistible to renew and to make wholeness manifest. When we are full of faith and cooperate with this restoring principle of our being, God's work of restoration never ceases its activity in us. He seeks always to restore harmony, strength, life, wholeness in that which He has created. Our holding thoughts like these and communing with the indwelling Presence in the silence gives to the healing Christ within the best possible opportunity to do His work quickly. If we could stay in harmony with the natural law at all times, our bodies, being self-renewing, would never wear out.

The Truth of Being

In his right relation, man is the inlet and the outlet of an everywhere present life, substance, and intelligence. He fits into the universal movement, but does not control or determine it. He must bring himself into harmony with it. He must blend his life consciously with God-life, his intelligence with God-intelligence, and his body with the "Lord's body." Then and only then will he be in right relation with the universe. God-Mind is eternally, perfectly in order. We should not pray for Him to change to correspond with our human need, but rather mold our own consciousness according to His perfection. Spiritually, man is God's idea of Himself as He sees Himself in the ideal. Physically, man is the law executing that idea. We are all in mind related to that great creative Spirit that infuses its life into our minds and bodies when we turn our attention to it. We have mentally wandered away from this creative Spirit or Father-Mind and lost contact with its life-giving currents. Jesus made connection for us, and through Him we again begin to draw vitality from the great fountainhead.

We must learn to make the right use of what we have. Devotion to that which is highest and best, without neglect of the physical, will result in an awakening which will give us light and peace and freedom. By using right ideas, man can manifest any form or shape that he may desire. What is termed *life* has its source in an idea of action. What is termed *intelligence* has its source in an idea of knowing. All manifestations have their source in some idea in mind. The only limitation is negative thought of man's imaging.

57

Applying this reasoning to individual consciousness, we find just how man thinks his body into disease. Instead of basing his thought on what is true in the absolute of Being, he bases it on conditions as they appear in the formed realm about him, and the result is bodily discord in multitudinous shapes. When the patient catches the vision of his perfection in Spirit, healing is sure to result. His body may appear to be diseased, but this appearance soon changes to health. At no time should we let the appearance of disease deflect us from our purpose of knowing and applying Truth.

The way to establishing divine order in our lives is through the study and application of Truth principles. We as individuals lose health, peace of mind, or other desirable states by our failure to know how to identify ourselves with God the Father, to use His gifts to us, and to let Spirit express through all our faculties and powers. We must recognize God as omnipresent, as the very life from which we have our being, as the innate intelligence that is present in every cell and nerve of our body. Definite study and training are required for righteous expression of our threefold nature. If we would have the full, free use of our senses and our organs, we must get at the causes of the inharmonies, remove them, and establish a new and perfect pattern and plan of action. We do this by remembering that we are God's children, that He has created us perfect, and that there is a law established within us that will keep us unfolding harmoniously if we will but recognize it.

Question Helps

1. Define "constructive thought."
2. How is man a threefold being?
3. What is the function of affirmations?
4. Why is the correct spiritual viewpoint so important in spiritual healing?
5. How does man establish divine order in his life?

Personal Notes

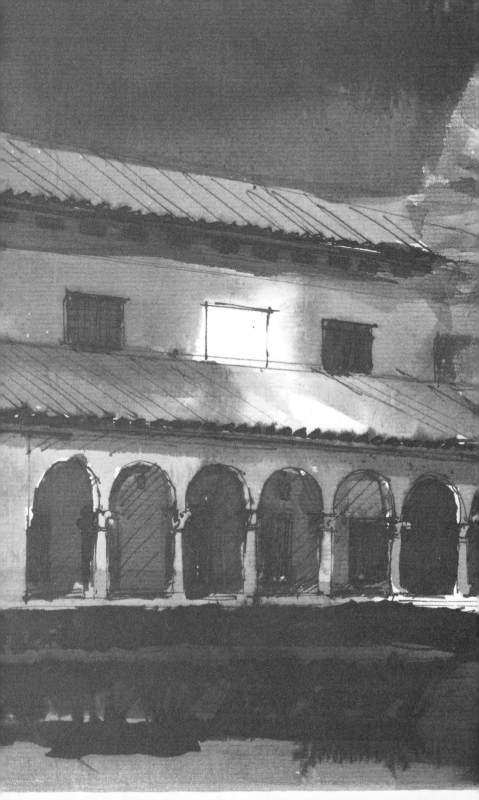

Mental Cause Revealed

Universal thought substance records and transcribes even the slightest vibration of thought. If we count health and disease as equal, the thought stuff of our minds will animate them with like potency. We will find ourselves believing that disease is just as real and far more catching than health.

Yet a moment's analysis of the relation between disease and health shows that health is the real, God-given condition, and disease the unreal, the abnormal, from which we are all seeking to escape. Truth not only shows the reality at the core of all things; it also shows that we shall never escape from the unreal so long as we allow our mental processes to give it power. If we deny disease as devoid of reality and affirm health as spiritual and abiding, Spirit will bear witness with our spirit and we will demonstrate health.

Distinguishing Truth and Error

Our subconscious mind controls all body functions whether we are asleep or awake, aware of them or not: breathing, heart action, circulation, elimination. The subconscious records all of what we think and believe, whether we want it to or not. We give it the orders; it carries them out. We must carefully choose what thoughts and emotions we want the subconscious to carry out. The conscious mind must learn to distinguish between truth and error, to recognize the falsehood of diseased conditions and not report them to the subconscious as "true." Wholeness and perfection are the only things that are true.

Your body receives vitalizing instructions from Spirit, but it accepts your personal suggestions also. When you tell it that it is tired, it believes you. You do not have to say "Body, you are tired," in so many words, but the very thought that you have in the back of your mind, the idea that your body is material and subject to weariness, means that you are making that suggestion to it.

Thoughts are things; they occupy space in the mental field. A healthy state of mind is achieved and maintained when the thinker willingly lets go the old thoughts and takes on the new. The action of the mind on the body is, in some of its aspects, similar to that of water on the earth. Living old thoughts over and over keeps the inlet of the new thoughts closed. Then begins crystallization.

A Change of Mind Pattern

We must learn to look to the mental man for causes. The physician takes it for granted that disease germs exist as an integral part of the natural world; the metaphysician sees disease germs as the manifested results of anger, revenge, jealousy, fear, impurity, and many other mind activities. A change of mind will change the character of a germ. Love, courage, strength, peace, and good will form good character and build bodily structures of a nature like these qualities of mind. If you think of yourself as anything less than the perfect child of the perfect Parent, you lower your thought standard and cut off the influx of thought from Divine Mind. "You, therefore, must be perfect, as your heavenly Father is perfect."

From ancestors, from the commonly accepted beliefs of the race, and from many other sources, error thoughts about God and man have been drawn to and stored in the subconscious, as have been error thoughts of the individual himself. After errors have become subconscious, they work themselves out in the body as disease, possibly long after the conscious mind has forgotten them. The natural balance of life forces in the body can be thrown off by negative emotions. These feelings can cause congestion in one part of the body, such as the congestion of a head cold resulting from a fear of cold air. We do not dispel anxiety, tension, depression, or fear without getting to the cause and overcoming it. This means a recognition on our part that negative emotions and feelings in us are the result of our sense of separation from God. The more we turn to God in prayer and establish ourselves in an awareness of oneness with Him, the more we feel balanced, poised, and at peace. God is always with us; we need only act on that knowledge and use our faith. Whatever the cause of the appearance of negation, turning the attention Godward with willingness to make such adjustments in daily living as are wise and loving toward the body will quickly relieve all strain and congestion and allow the free flow of life to renew nerves and structures. The body responds to changes of mind, and when this is accompanied by truly wise living habits, the conformity to true ideas of life, power, love, substance, and intelligence will renew it and make it whole.

Every form in the universe, every function, all action, all substance—all these have a thinking part that is receptive to and controllable by man. Material science has observed that every molecule has three things: intelligence, substance, and action. It knows where it wants to go, it has form, and it moves. Man can control matter by means of this intelligence. Man can dissolve things by denying their existence, and he can build them by affirming their presence. If man affirms the spirituality of his being, it will manifest in his perfect body; if he believes in and affirms the material, he will be burdened with a material body, subject to physical ills. It is widely held today that a great majority of the ills to which the flesh seems heir are emotionally induced. We poison ourselves with worry and excessive concern over work, health, loved ones, prosperity or lack thereof. When we indulge in prolonged periods of worry, resentment, tension, or fear, we are specifically inviting physical congestion and illness. We usually do not have long to wait before our invitation is accepted.

We can actually see or feel the effect of fear and hatred by stomach cramps, fogginess of vision, shortness of breath, and a pounding heart.

Dwell on God

"Trust in the Lord, and do good; . . . Take delight in the Lord and he will give you the desires of your heart." In other words: stop thinking about and worrying about the conditions that happen around you and to you, and start thinking about God. Let Him stabilize and control the attitudes and reactions that happen *in* you. Don't fight apparent error, injustice, darkness. Instead, return to the principle. Don't dwell on the problem; dwell on God.

If a man thinks about the power of sin (thinks in error), he builds up and gives force to that belief until it engulfs him in its whirlpool of thought substance. He forgets his spiritual origin and sees only the human. He thinks of himself as a sinner, rather than as the image and likeness of God.

Man also sees the law of sowing and reaping, and he fears his sins and their results. Then fear of the divine law is added to his burdens. The way out of this maze of ignorance, sin, and sickness is through man's understanding of his real being, and then the forgiving or giving up of all thoughts of the reality of sin and its effects in the body.

Any thought that is not based on the eternal reality, Truth, really has no existence at all, so if we believe in disease, we are believing in something that has no substance or reality. When we replace that belief with a conviction that we are one with the Father, we will soon be expressing His perfect health.

God is never absent from us. He is constantly taking form in our lives according to the exact pattern of our words, thoughts, and actions. Just as soon as we bring our words and our expectations up to the measure of God's love for us, just that soon will we demonstrate.

64

We have the power to change conditions, to express our Godlike nature. Keeping the attention centered in the Christ Mind, we are able to see beyond appearances to the impulse of spirit, which is always urging us in our efforts to make use of what God has given. To the degree that we let Christ be lifted up, in the same degree shall we rid ourselves of that which may have been pronounced incurable.

The Whole Man

True healing is threefold: spiritual, mental, and physical. A person cannot be truly whole if one of these parts is ailing, as all are inextricably linked. Man has been treated too long as a dichotomy or a trichotomy. He is led to think of himself as three or more distinct entities. He must go to a doctor for treatment of his body, to a psychologist or psychiatrist for treatment of mental or emotional problems, and to a minister, rabbi, or priest for treatment of problems of the soul or spirit. There is a great need for communication among all three areas of healing, for none of these aspects can be treated without affecting the others.

Man is one, not three. Spirit, mind, and body are not different entities, requiring specialists for their care and treatment. The healers who are most successful are those who deal with the whole man. These include doctors who encourage supplementary prayer and spiritual treatment, as well as practitioners of spiritual healing who do not resist supplementary medical treatment for those for whom they are praying, but who accept it as an expedient sometimes made necessary by certain states of consciousness.

It remains, however, that the greatest healing treatment known to man is based on the words, "Thou dost keep him in perfect peace, whose mind is stayed on thee." You will have perfect balance of all the natural healing functions of your body if your mind is stayed on God in a consciousness of love, faith, and peace.

Spiritual Viewpoint

Joyous, radiant health is the result of the right *spiritual* viewpoint, the continuous purposeful effort to unfold the faculties and *soul* qualities, and the daily recognition of the *body* as the temple of God and the structure that Spirit and soul are building. All these prompt us to give careful attention to the needs of the system. Observance of the law is threefold: spiritual, keeping a person assured of his God-given freedom from all anxiety, worry, fear, and lack; mental, giving him the intelligence that enables him always to do that which promotes health and success; physical, establishing those habits which keep him making the right use of all his faculties, powers, and life energy and substance. A person cannot cultivate one and neglect the others, for weakness, sickness, inharmony, or imperfection in the organism is the result of some failure to identify oneself with God, the divine Source, and to understand how to lay hold of and express one's inheritance of spiritual powers; some limitation in the soul's development of its riches; or some ignorance of the body's requirements and disregard of the divine law of life and health.

One who remembers and lives by the spiritual promises of the law of health will not worry, seek to manage other people's affairs, or neglect to feed his own soul with that which is necessary to keep it unfolding Christward.

One who is aware of the mental side of his health seeks to keep himself free from the limitations of the race mind, the opinions and demands of others, the depressions and hurried attitudes that keep the Christ ideas from finding perfect expression through his thoughts and acts.

One who is determined that his physical life shall show forth the peace and order of the spiritual reality and the divine intelligence is considerate of his body and careful in his demands upon it. He sees to it that he understands the physical requirements and that he meets these every day.

It is well to understand where one has been making mistakes—judging by appearances, accepting illusions, working contrary to Principle, using the faculties in ways not intended by the Creator. These mistakes and misuses of one's God-given faculties are the cause of human inharmonies. The change of causes also changes the effects.

When the individual keeps his mind in tune with God-Mind, he knows constant harmony, order, success, and health. By following the teaching of Jesus Christ and seeking guidance of the Most High, he does not leave room for a negative thought to enter.

The Creator is continually doing His work of restoration throughout His creation, especially in every man and every woman, for He puts all His children into the world to manifest His perfection. When we learn how to cooperate with this all-powerful Spirit of restoration, nothing can stand in the way of our manifesting the health that belongs to us by divine right.

Natural Rhythm and Harmony

Resolve to become one with God through Christ. Harmonize yourself with Him, and all your world will be in harmony. Be on the alert to see harmony everywhere. Do not magnify seeming differences. Do not keep up any petty divisions, but continually declare the one universal harmony. Perfect health comes from getting back into harmony with God's plan by getting our thoughts in order. When we use an affirmation for healing we should lift our thoughts above the sense world so that we do not dwell upon the negative conditions that we are trying to dispel. We should let our creative thoughts work in the realm of spiritual perfection so that they may bring us back into harmony with God's spiritual creation. When this is done our healing takes place.

In harmony and rhythm lies the secret of life and health. Every atom of being is thrilling with rhythmic vibration. Measured movements are detected in every department of life. When breathing is natural, it is performed rhythmically. All natural movement is orderly and regular. To the person who finds rhythm and surrenders himself to it, the natural expression is ease, charm, and freedom, whether he is speaking, acting, singing, walking, or swimming. He who violates rhythmic order interferes with harmonious action and reaction, thereby cutting himself off from the source of energy and substance. The man who is in rhythm with the natural forces has the force of all vibrations—those of the tides, of the change of season, of day and night—working with him.

Declare daily that your spiritual life and world, your mental life and world, your physical life and world are unified and that you are expressing harmoniously the ideas of the Christ Mind on these three planes. Know that your everyday physical life can and should be inspired and happy and purposeful, not strained and tense, and that it is never necessary to do that which is harmful or weakening to any of the functions or organs in accomplishing what is right. As you practice mentally seeing God's plan in your life, you will find that you are better poised, that you will do just the right thing, and that your body will be healthy.

The Peace of God

The first step in manifesting health is to become still. Divine Mind is serene, orderly, placid, while sense mind is turbulent, discordant, and violent. The best of us are subject to crosscurrents of worry that interfere with the even flow of God's thoughts into our consciousness. Jesus warned His followers not to be anxious about what they should eat, drink, or wear. There is a natural law whose chief purpose is to take care of the human family, but the divine order of creative Mind must be observed by man before he can receive the benefits of his natural inheritance.

Metaphysicians find that when they refuse to let thoughts of worry, anxiety, or other distraction act in their minds, they gradually establish an inner quietness that finally merges into a great peace. This is the "peace of God, which passes all understanding." When this peace is attained, the individual gets inspiration and revelation direct from infinite Mind. This inner peace can be attained whenever outer thoughts are stilled, in sleep, in meditation, or in profound relaxation.

Instinctive Wholeness

It is our right and natural state to be well and strong. People will try almost anything that promises to give them more life and vitality, because they have an instinctive belief in health. While all of us desire life and health, sometimes this desire is clouded over and even superseded by our desire for love and understanding, by our need to feel cared for, by our desire for attention. If we have been surrounded by much love and attention because of illness and have become dependent on others, our desire for healing and for a return to normal, responsible living may be weakened. Without our being consciously aware of it, we may have accepted sickness as our way of life. Some persons may be ill because it gains them those things that they feel they cannot get in any other way: attention and care, getting away from too much pressure or work, avoiding something that they do not want to do. These persons have invited their illness and hold to it without being consciously aware of doing so. But in their inmost self they are in conflict, for the desire to live and to stand strong and free is greater than the desire for ease, comfort, and sympathy.

69

The Will to Live

The will to live is in us all, and we are not happy or at peace with ourselves when we are not expressing this will of God in us. Though everyone else praises us for endurance and patience under suffering, we want more than patience and endurance; we want life, the abundant life that Jesus promised.

There are many reasons that a person should be inclined to develop a consciousness of sickness. He may have been overprotected as a child. Some households are very germ- and disease-oriented, with much talk about disease and physical dangers. There is much publicity in the media about various disorders such as headaches and colds. Discussion about so-called "hereditary diseases" sets the stage for their later development. We should take care not to dwell on a particular fear or disease, for thought can bring into manifestation just what we fear. Do not claim disease or the inclination to disease for your own.

How many times have we been told to be careful—careful not to get our feet wet, careful not to sit in drafts, careful not to get close to people who aren't well, careful of what we eat, careful to get the right amount of sleep. Medical science continuously investigates ways to prevent sickness. Immunizations have been developed; corrective surgery is done; weight reduction is urged; exercise is encouraged—all as preventive measures. More people today than ever before are trying to eat right, adding vitamins and minerals to their diets. More of us are thinking about prevention on the physical side, but we haven't thought much about prevention from the spiritual point of view. It is easy, simple, and comprehensive to consider spiritual wholeness the goal.

If we need healing, what is important: temperature, pulse rate, and so on, or the healing? Where we place the emphasis of our thoughts and attention makes a difference in healing. Those who treat the sick say that sometimes their patients get so enmeshed in symptoms, in pains, in how they feel today as compared with yesterday, that they withdraw into a circumscribed world where the body and its demands receive their undivided attention.

Temple of God

How differently we feel when we think of our bodies as the temple of the living God, as the actual dwelling place of the Holy Spirit! How differently we feel when we realize that there is only one life, God-life, and that this life flows through us, a mighty, healing, purifying, cleansing stream. Such thoughts are so inspiring and life-giving that we do not even want to talk about anything but life. We no longer attach importance to every little twinge or ache or pain. We declare life, we hold to life, we express life. And in doing so, we are healed!

Question Helps

1. How is a healthy state of mind achieved and maintained?
2. "Negative emotions throw off the natural balance of life forces." Explain.
3. What can happen if a man thinks about the power of sin?
4. Explain why true healing is threefold.
5. How should one use an affirmation for harmony?
6. What is the first step in manifesting health?

Personal Notes

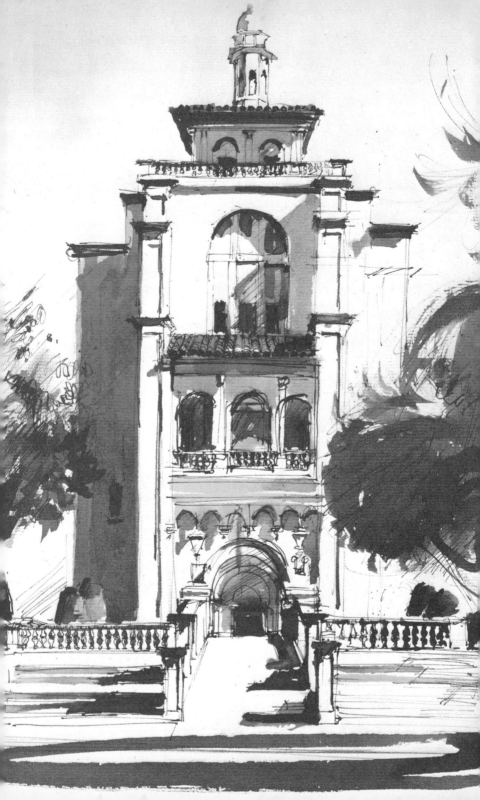

Live Wisely and Well

Remember that there is a friendly, loving intelligence in your body watching over it night and day, keeping it in repair and seeing that its organs are functioning smoothly. This intelligence never sleeps on the job, for whether you are awake or asleep it works on unceasingly, mending torn tissues, cleansing your blood, eliminating waste, knitting bones if necessary, digesting food, and making chemical fluids. It is a force that cleanses, lubricates, and coordinates the parts of your body and also protects it from destructive forces from within.

This wise "repairman" is a silent agent of God in you, carrying out God's loving command that you be a living soul and have dominion over all the Earth. But do not forget that it needs your cooperation in order to do its best work. If you worry, overeat, dissipate, or think destructive thoughts, you may tear down your body faster than it can be built up.

Free Your Body

Realizing clearly that your body forces are a part of God's plan will promote harmony and health in your body. Practice daily putting all the parts and functions of your body into God's hands and you will help Him to help you. Free your body from your worries and fears and from inherited ideas concerning the weaknesses and disease to which it is supposed to be subject.

Scientists tell us that the body is self-renewing and that if it were properly nourished and its functions were not interfered with, they would go on indefinitely. Prayer acts as a balance upon the thought and the body forces. When the body forces are equalized, there can be no anemia in one part of the body and no congestion or blush in another. Prayer relieves and removes chronic adverse thoughts. The thought that produces a blush or a blanched condition of the face for a moment or two may be of little consequence but the thought of anger, jealousy, revenge, or discouragement that could hold a vital organ in its grip for months or years could do serious damage to the health.

God's method of operating in us is purely this: His work takes place when we no longer set up adverse thoughts as barriers. Your reactions to the little situations in life make you either healthy or unhealthy in mind and in body. If you are inclined to resist and to fight in mind the situations you have to meet, you will find that you set up a state of tension in the body. If you are unfriendly toward the persons you meet, your mental attitude causes an adverse state in your physical condition. If you are loving in your reactions, your physical body receives a loving blessing. There is nothing external about these reactions; they are entirely under our control. We can think whatever we desire and thus can train ourselves to react wholesomely and healthily to all situations.

Do not resist outside conditions or fight them mentally. The only result of your resistance will be tension and physical disorder.

Quiet Miracles

We need not be forced to seek Truth by some harsh experience in life, but we can start now through prayer and meditation to put our lives and our thoughts in order. In this way, severe experiences will be avoided. Spiritual awareness—and with it, order of body and mind—grows steadily by means of daily prayer and meditation.

The quiet miracles of prayer take many forms: releasing the pressure of mental and emotional tensions in some form of confession, by confiding repressed thoughts and feelings to a doctor, friend, or counselor, or by "writing a letter to God"; silent communion with nature; physical exercise; some creative hobby such as woodcarving, clay modeling, handicrafts; or service to others less fortunate than ourselves. All these activities serve to take us "out of ourselves," to shift our forces and enable us to touch the healing power of God. All these miracles of prayer are based on giving in creative and constructive ways. To pray for another is healing to the self.

Prayer opens the way for us to draw on the infinite reservoir of God-Mind, to bring into manifestation that which is already ours. Prayer is getting in touch with Spirit, the method of overcoming error thoughts. Prayer liberates the energies pent up in mind and body and enables them to be put to use in constructive ways.

Praying Life into Expression

To acquire the mind that is always open to Spirit, we must be persistent in prayer. The one who prays for healing must persist in this prayer until the walls of resistance are broken down and the healing currents are tuned in. "The prayer of faith will save the sick man, and the Lord will raise him up." When the mind becomes trustful and confident, it is in harmony with creative Mind, and its force flows to us in accordance with the law of like attracting like.

The agonizing, supplicating, begging prayer is not answered, because the thoughts are so turbulent that Divine Mind cannot reach the pleader. Jesus prayed with a confident assurance that what He wanted would be granted, and this should serve as a model for our own prayer.

We need to stir up and quicken our senses. Our organism has been asleep from disuse and lack of vital interest in living—not merely in eating, drinking, sleeping, and being entertained, but in the essential issues that have to do with bringing ourselves into the full-rounded Jesus Christ expression of life. If a person would be healed and would keep getting younger, more vigorous and alert, and ready for what the times demand of him, he would wake up and get out of the rut, change his habits, appropriate the life elements in food, in sunshine, and especially in Truth statements.

Not only must we believe, but we must *act*. We must not only perceive an idea; we must also give it form by infusing into it the substance of our living faith. There are two sides to every proposition, the image and the expression, just as the Lord God formed the image man out of the ground and breathed into his nostrils the breath of life. So each one of us must not only see the image of his desires as a theory but he must also form it into a living, breathing thing through every motive and act of his life. That is, if we have an idea, we must act just as if it were part of our lives. There must be an actual imaging of perfect health in our consciousness before we shall ever see that idea realized.

Manifest Substance

Spirit within is the quickening, adjusting, harmonizing force. We must agree to think health, to bless the body, and to express that which causes all the functions of the organisms to work perfectly. But Spirit must have substance through which to manifest! You must provide the manifest substance and life elements in proper food, drink, sunshine, and air. Without these, Spirit would have no vehicle, for these are drawn from the outside.

Pay especial attention to living habits. Bathe with the idea of opening all the millions of little doors of the skin to let out used-up materials and to let in sunshine and its energy. Eat with the understanding that you are providing God-given materials which the inner intelligence will use to nourish, cleanse, and renew all of your body every day. There are foods for the muscle tissues, others for the blood, others for the glands, for skin and hair and nails and brain and eyes. Grown-ups and children can do without homes of their own, without good furniture, without cars, without many of the luxuries that have grown to be everyday habits with many. But all of them, large or small, need time for quiet and for well-planned meals and for attention to the little things—little in themselves, but necessary to health. Do not overtax the body by giving forth more than you have taken the time and the quietness to receive. It is best to listen within and take the hint to relax and recoup when you hear it. Do not drive the body beyond its comfortable capacities. You are eternally one with your Source and Creator, so it is just a matter of getting still, calm, and serene, with your thought away for a while from all the outer activities, and of opening the way for the mighty and abundant inflow of Spirit that vitalizes, invigorates, and renews every part of mind, heart, and body. Unlimited as the infinite Provider is as our resource, we must still the restless mortal in order to receive; then the inner substance will fill our relaxed and receptive organism to brimming.

Love Balances

It is possible to drive oneself beyond what the soul and body can stand up under, if wisdom and love do not prompt. One may lean too much toward intellectual activities—drawing and holding too much of the blood and nerve energy in the upper part of the body and causing congestion and depletion. One may devote oneself so wholly to those things, good in themselves, which require undivided attention and nerve strain that the playtimes for the body which permit relaxation and renewal are neglected. One can engage in so-called "spiritual work" to the point of losing one's health. In order to benefit humanity most we must each one see to it that we are fair to ourselves and that we live a life that increases our power and strength and health—that is, a balanced life.

Unity emphasizes control of the physical by the spiritual. The real control is in living according to the perfect pattern and law. It is not spiritual thought that prompts one to abuse the body in any way. It is not spiritual desire that allows one to eat when there is no need of food or to partake of food elements that are not what the body requires at the time. It is not spiritual thought that causes one to worry, to become tense, or to drive the body in the effort to gain intellectually.

Let Life Flow

When negative attitudes of mind and heart cause depression, physical inharmony, and a feeling of lack and worry, a quiet hour for study and prayer will flood the soul with an entirely new light and peace. You will begin to relax and to allow the abundant life and wonderful love of God to flow freely through you, restoring order and health. You will see your affairs in a different way, and the inner assurance that God is providing, directing, and prompting will give you great peace. You will invite and lay hold of your own individual God-given resources, for in truth God does provide for you, and your blessings are not dependent upon others. You can use your own faculties and powers and bring forth that which you require—and you will be the better for this purposeful living.

Keep on praying for faith, because it is through prayer that you develop all your wonderful qualities. Drugs will not do the healing; they are just something tangible on which to place your attention while God is doing His work of restoration. "I am the Lord, your healer." If you need something visible to the human eye upon which to place your faith, it is better to study dietetics and to give your body the right kinds of food. Right thinking and right eating go hand in hand in keeping one healthy.

There is no reason why the machinery in our body temples should wear out, because the Creator is still on the job, building up and renewing His temple to the extent that we permit. When we cooperate by thinking habitually in terms of eternal life, eternal youth, ever-increasing strength, and perfect health, we are renewed moment by moment. God is constantly renewing and revitalizing every human being.

Never Too Late

Jesus said, "Whatever you ask in prayer, you will receive, if you have faith." Learn to give thanks in the realization that you are already healed. It is never too late to pray. No matter what the need, the condition, the problem, it is never too late for God's power to act, for His perfect work to be done in mind, body, and affairs. Do not let yourself believe that there is ever a time when God cannot help you.

Jesus, in the healing He performed, never questioned the power of God to heal. He said, "With God all things are possible." He knew that it was not too late to heal the man born blind; it was not too late to heal the man who had been crippled for thirty-eight years. He spoke the word of life. He knew that where there was faith there was answered prayer.

It is never too late to begin again, to put old failure and negation behind. It is never too late to begin again with a completely new attitude, to live with Christ in newness of life.

Paul said: "And God is able to provide you with every blessing in abundance, so that you may always have enough of everything and may provide in abundance for every good work." Paul is telling us (and he proved it in his own experience) that when there is a limitation that appears to be a handicap, the action of Spirit is greater in and around the limitation than at any other point. This is why handicaps can actually be helpful. The handicapped person is blessed with a focus of infinite intelligence and energy working in him to compensate and to lead him beyond the problem to normalcy and achievement. He may (and often does) allow the problem to turn him to self-pity, to discouragement, and to an experience of limitation, but if he knows the Truth and is willing to let the activity of God's grace flow through him, then nothing is impossible to him.

Seed of Advantage

We are here to develop and to grow, and we must work with what we have, no matter how mean it may seem to us. In every adversity there lies the seed of an equivalent advantage. You are not limited except by your own thought. Do not allow another's appraisal of your situation to justify feelings of insufficiency. Do not judge by the appearance of your negative condition, but know that it can be overcome. Do not accept the worldly appraisal of possibilities; do not limit yourself, for therein lies the problem.

Many famous and successful men started out in a "handicapped" state: Napoleon was short and born extremely poor; Demosthenes had a speech impediment; Norman Vincent Peale suffered with feelings of insecurity, shyness, and inferiority; Abraham Lincoln had little education and was very poor; Beethoven became deaf. Men like these demonstrate that handicaps need not and should not be a barrier to success. A handicap can cause a person to become aware that there exists something mightier than the circumstance of his limitation. Handicaps are not to be accepted as punishment or the "will of God." The burdens of man—poverty, sickness, inharmony, wars—are not God's will, nor are they the work of some satanic force of evil. They become burdens because man gives power to lack in his thinking—lack of prosperity, lack of health, lack of harmony, lack of peace.

Do not accept a limiting concept of God. His will is for the perfect health, perfect success, perfect life of all

His creations. God's will for you now is for you to succeed, regardless of the experiences or seeming limitations with which you find yourself bound. You can succeed in spite of your adversity, and, more than you may now realize, your chances of success could even be enhanced because of it.

The handicap itself is not the problem. The cause of difficulty is the person's *attitude* toward the handicap. He limits himself by admitting the existence of the handicap. A man can be crippled only in his mind.

Abundant Compensation

We may profit from difficulty. If life is too easy, serene, without problems, we are not prodded to grow and to develop. Use your limitation not as an excuse for failure, but as a tool for growth. God wills only that we grow and unfold, that we express our potential. He will not allow you to be challenged beyond your innate ability to overcome. He will, through the handicap or the limitation, become a concentrated activity and motivation that seeks a means of compensating a way of success.

Compensation is a well-known phenomenon in the field of medicine. There have been numerous cases where one kidney was damaged, and the other increased in size and did the work of two. If one eye is weak, the other becomes much stronger. Blind persons usually have well-developed senses of touch, smell, and hearing. Man, physically weak among animals, uses his brain and material weapons to advance. Thus an apparent weakness often leads to the development of a strength. The love of God for us is so great, and the longing of God to perfect Himself in and through us is so relentless, that we never receive the full harvest of our sowing of error. We always receive a little more of good than we sow. There exists an all-sufficiency equal to, and surpassing, every challenge.

Question Helps

1. How does prayer relieve chronic adverse thoughts?
2. Why is balanced life so important?
3. What should one do when negative attitudes cause depression?
4. Why is it never too late to pray?
5. "Man is not limited except by his own thoughts." Explain.
6. How can one profit from difficulty?

Personal Notes

The Body Temple

There is a divine law of mind action that we may conform to and that will always bring beneficial results. There is also a physical side to the operation of this divine law. The body and its needs must have our consideration. We must not drive the body or neglect its normal needs.

This body is the result of our use of God-given faculties and powers. We have needed such a temple, and the soul has built it. Sometimes we fail to remember that the temple is for the use of the Holy Spirit. Our bodies are very necessary members of the trinity that makes up our being. We would not be a complete being without it. We are spirit, soul, and body, three parts of the divine-man idea, in one. These three must become unified in order that we may become a perfect expression of God's ideal man. By lifting up our bodies, seeing it as Spirit substance instead of matter, we help to unify it with our true spiritual nature.

Evidently, the individual soul has felt the need of just such an Earth home as the body temple. We are to realize that the body, free from the inharmonies and weaknesses imposed on it through error, is a part of God's plan of life.

A thing is not less spiritual because it has taken form and weight and color. The thing that might be termed "material" is the misconception or unwise combination of thoughts and elements that produces an undesirable result. Spirit becomes manifest in man's expression of what God gives.

Divine Ideas

Our religious lives, heretofore, has led us to feel that our thoughts and our emotions were all that was necessary to our spiritual experience, that the body was to be regarded as of little consequence and as really not responsive to the finer things of Spirit. What we must strive to remember, however, is that our bodies are more than flesh, blood, and bone. The body is an expression of the divine ideas of life, substance, and intelligence. If the body did not have intelligence, it could not repair cuts in its skin and knit together its broken bones. If it did not have intelligence, it could not operate the wonderful laboratory that digests its food and turns it into flesh, blood, bone, hair, energy, brains, and so forth. Without intelligence it could not keep our heart beating and our blood circulating even while we sleep.

Learn to affirm: "I do not own my body: I am body. I do not own my soul: I am soul. I do not own my spirit: I am Spirit. And these three are one."

Oneness with the Father

Jesus called the body the temple of God. He said that He and the Father were one. If the two are one, then there is no separation; if they are one, then they are one in the same body. Paul told us that God "does not dwell in houses made with hands," and that "God's Spirit dwells in you." If we accept our oneness with the Father, if we believe that He does dwell within us, then we will start taking better care of these physical temples, our bodies. We know that God has to express through us. This is the reason that we must keep our minds, bodies, and emotions as sound and healthy as possible—so that we can be a fit channel for His expression.

We should consider how marvelous the body is, how it functions with little or no direction from us, intricately and perfectly. We should develop sensible habits that help rather than hinder it in its marvelous work. Learn to appreciate your body! Praise and bless it, for it is truly a work of God.

Bless the Body

Sometimes, the soul gets so anxious about what it wishes to do that it tends to neglect the body. This is not fair to the body nor to those who must take care of the body when it is neglected. Our first duty, then, is to bless our bodies and to get our thoughts right about it, to praise its wonderful work, to learn what its needs are and to arrange for supplying them.

We sometimes become too ambitious, somewhere in the recesses of the soul, and starve the precious body temple. Then come hard experiences, blessings in disguise. For God is there in that body, and He will not let the soul continue to neglect the body. Suffering is one of the means of drawing the attention of the soul back to its temple. The Christ Mind can and will direct the soul in taking up its wonderful work in the body that it may continue to have this necessary vehicle of expression.

To the present time the followers of Jesus have been told by spiritual leaders that He taught the immortality of the soul only. But now it is revealed that He immortalized His body and said, "Follow me." It was man's sins that brought death to his body, and his redemption must include the healing of the body. When the mind is healed of its sins the body will respond. "Your body is a temple of the Holy Spirit within you, which you have from God."

So we find as we study and apply the doctrine of Jesus that the body must be included. Faith in the omnipresent pure substance precipitates substance in the body, and we are transformed.

Visible Vibration of Spirit

Truth students often entertain thoughts of conflict between the medical and spiritual approaches to healing, but there should be no conflict. They act as if they think that doctors and medicine represent some sort of evil force. We must remember that life is both spiritual and physical. The physical is simply the visible vibration of the Spirit, and the life that is Spirit permeates every living thing.

The teaching of Unity seeks to challenge us to come up higher, to press on to the goal of our own divine perfection. We should make every possible attempt to meet our needs on the highest possible level, and to "put away childish things," such as habitual dependence on drugs, stimulants, and physical treatment. We should not make the mistake, however, of trying to make a child into an adult overnight. We should take one step at a time, in patience, and even if we cannot get up and walk immediately, we can keep our eyes on the goal while crawling forward.

Principle is infinite, but we can demonstrate only at the level of our faith and consciousness. It is good to go carefully forward and to achieve what we are capable of achieving. We may not be able to feed a multitude of five thousand, but we can provide food for our own family.

Healing Agents

A spiritual counselor is often asked such questions as: "Should I have the operation the doctor advises, or should I go all the way with prayer?" "I am a diabetic, but I want to follow the way of prayer. Should I refuse to take my insulin?" The counselor cannot (and certainly should not attempt to) answer these questions for the student. The answer is within the student's own consciousness. By honest self-examination, he must seek the course that is right for him. If he finds within himself a calm and fearless realization of God as his perfect health, then no one should try to dissuade him from his determination to go all the way with prayer. He can be healed, even if there are those who say the odds are insurmountable. On the other hand, if even after praying about it, he continues to experience deep-seated fear (and there is no kidding oneself about this) then it may be that he is not yet ready to "walk on the water," to go forward on the next level of consciousness. His prayer might well be answered with guidance to employ some form of assistance in addition to prayer treatment. A good statement used by one Unity teacher is this: "Go first to God; go next to man as God directs." Wherever and however the healing energy is activated within the body temple and the healing life is induced into harmonious expression, it is good. There are times when the individual needs and should have all the help he can receive.

Renewing Power

Men of science (and this certainly includes the profession of medicine) have often been pictured as being completely materialistic, if not atheistic, in attitude, rejecting any concept of spiritual healing. Yet fundamental to the medical practitioner is a factor upon which he bases all his efforts: the healing power of nature. He accepts without question the concept that health is from within and does not have to be manufactured in the outer. He knows that he is not really a healer. Nature is the healer, and he simply cooperates through his understanding of nature's laws. In all his work, the doctor depends upon this healing power, the renewing power of life itself.

If some outward help is strongly indicated, do not let your prejudice against material help restrain you from doing what, in your highest and most practical understanding, you believe to be best. If you have a sliver in your finger, it is easier to pull it out with a pair of tweezers than to "think" it out, and common sense dictates the former course. If you have a dental cavity, and your seeking of God's help in meeting the need is not accompanied by a demonstrable improvement, it is the part of wisdom to have the tooth cared for by the very best possible dentist, looking upon him as an agent of God in your healing. Then try to keep your thoughts and life activities—which include keeping your teeth clean—in such good order that you will not need further fillings.

Most students need encouragement, not in employing material helps when good sense indicates their use, but rather in freeing themselves from too great a dependence upon them. It is probably in these agencies only secondarily, and sometimes not at all, but certainly in the patient's response to the diverse methods that healing is attained. And even though faith is a great factor in human response, some of these methods are effective where no active faith in the afflicted person is discernible. They are effective, apparently, in the degree that they act as a stimulus to the innate restorative powers within the patient's organism.

Faith Heals

As a rule, material remedies work because people believe in them. The dominant force in healing is faith. "According to your faith be it done to you." "Your faith has saved you." "Be it done for you as you have believed." It is your faith that heals you, no matter if you use a material remedy as a "prop" or not. Your healing comes with the spiritualization of your mind, with the adjustment of your belief to the pure reason of God-knowing. The Christ faith, dwelling in man, blots out the errors of sins of his past; his recognition of the Truth of his being, through unity with his Father, is bodied forth as perfection, and according to his faith he becomes whole.

Release Concern

Do not worry or feel guilty if you have failed so far to heal yourself through prayer. We are all on the path to perfection, but we must move forward one step at a time. Do not dwell on your apparent "failure," but remedy it through medical means if necessary (such as

88

wearing glasses to correct shortsidedness). This will relieve any strain or worry about the condition and free your energy for better works. Not only that, but you may find that the worrisome condition improves as soon as you release your concern about it. One Unity teacher values his own glasses very much, for he finds that they not only help him to read better, but they also help him to be understanding and tolerant when he meets an individual who finds it necessary to accept his healing at a level below the highest potential. Do not resist a condition such as imperfect sight; do not fight and make that the purpose of your existence. Release it, and give thanks for the optometrist's skill to correct it. Do what you can, start where you are, use what understanding and faith you now have. Go as far as your faith will carry you. Through the constant exercise of faith, you will be surprised at how far you can go. Do not chastize yourself for "failing" or be concerned that others will think you are falling short. It is false pride to keep up an appearance of Truth for others to see only.

Divine Liberation

In the beginning of spiritual unfoldment, divine understanding may seem to be operating in a dim light, to be clouded, indistinct, indecisive. But within each of us is a spiritual law that, if we industriously affirm it, will develop in us the power to use the attributes of God and to understand their place and their work. It is not always easy to live up to our good resolutions or to demonstrate healing. Often we have been sincere in making the resolutions, but the old mental conceptions formed by limited understanding resist the new inspiration; they try to hold their ground. This resistance causes a letting down in consciousness. It takes patience, perseverance, and industry to remold the perceptive and directive power of the mind. While the process may be slow, it is sure if we keep on. Our problem is to gather enough energy, power, love, wisdom, and pure light within to enable us to breathe divine liberation into the soul, into the very flesh; to arouse sufficient power to lift up the whole consciousness until we see with an understanding heart.

Timeless Spirit of Health

There is no time in Spirit, and its work begins just as soon as we turn our thoughts toward God for healing. If there seems to be a delay in the manifestation of healing, do not be concerned. The delay merely shows that you need to pray for a better understanding of the healing law in order that you may live in more perfect accord with it. Faithful work in daily prayer and meditation and affirmation invariably will bring good results. Do not dwell on the desired result, but concentrate on the building of a better faith and a clearer understanding. Think about the Source; the results will come naturally.

God is, eternal and everlasting. In Spirit we are already healed, so time passed is a misconception. Do not worry at all about the time element; let it go. Do not expect or dread a delay. If healing does not come immediately, persist in the application of your prayers. Release all fear, and trust in God. Listen within after praying, for God may then give you guidance which you might miss if you are not receptive.

There is no limitation on God's healing power, no delay, no time involved. If we are not healed instantly, the delay and the limitation can only be in us, in our unawareness of our oneness with eternal, healing life, now in the instant we voice our prayer. There is God-life and God-intelligence in every cell of our bodies. The body is responsive to our every thought about it. When we are ill, we are aware of the aches, the pains, the things that seem wrong, and we burden the body further by our fears and nagging worries concerning it.

90

We should be careful to direct our thoughts away from these areas and instead affirm life and strength in our every part.

Continual Renewal

True healing is not determined by time as we know it. True healing does not depend on the nature of the disease or its duration. True healing is of God, from God, and is the return, in a flash, in an instant—in the eternity that is God's time—to the perfection in which we were created. God created us as perfectly good; He still sees us in our perfection. He does not see the illness, the hurts, the imperfections. His love sees only the perfect child of God. The creative Spirit that breathed us into life in the first place is continually pouring life through us, continually renewing us, continually healing us. We need to dwell not on our symptoms or on the negativity of conditions, but to know and to affirm God's vitalizing, freeing life. In a very real sense we are renewed continually—mentally, physically, and spiritually.

We may understand that we can think new thoughts and that we can attain new spiritual insight, but we may not be able to accept the idea of newness for our bodies. If we have some condition that is termed chronic, we often fail to think in terms of newness and healing of the condition. We more often pray to be able to live with our illness, and this only hinders our healing.

If we desire to demonstrate health, we must order our lives rightly, for if it is not so ordered, mental and physical discord will ensue. This applies to all that we think and do. Everything must be brought into order. If we affirm prosperity, that too must be brought into orderly relation to the rest of our thinking. We may be declaring life and prosperity and at the same time be holding some disorganizing thought. This will produce inharmony in body and affairs. Lack of orderly arrangement of thoughts is responsible for many delayed demonstrations of healing.

Question Helps

1. Why is man's body a temple?
2. How does faith heal?
3. There should be no conflict between the medical and spiritual approaches to healing. Explain why.
4. Why is faith the dominant force in healing?
5. What should one do when the manifestation of healing is delayed?
6. Explain the importance of order in demonstrating health.

Personal Notes

The Myth of Aging

God-Mind rests in a perpetual realization of health, and that which seems to be sickness does not exist in Truth. There is no such thing as a "disease" or incurable condition in the system. These activities, weaknesses, or abnormalities to which the medical profession gives names are but the efforts of the God-given inner intelligence to deal with conditions that the individual has produced by his failure to recognize himself as the perfect child of God and to live by the divine law of life. Anything that does not measure up to the Christ pattern of perfection can be changed. Anything that the idea of God-Mind, expressing in the mind of man, has not produced can be dissolved into nothingness by the correct application of spiritual thought and the resultant spiritual action—and this includes illness.

Disease is not something of itself; it is only a condition of consciousness. When someone who has had a doctor diagnose his case comes to us, we ask him to turn deliberately from the doctor's opinions and cease to think of the name he gave to the condition that existed at the time of the examination. We ask him to cast out and forget the assumption that this condition could not be changed and done away with utterly. We take care not to name the apparent disorder, for to name something defines it and gives it reality, hence power. It is well for anyone, when beginning healing prayers, first to deny the medical name of the seeming inharmony. It is not good to call inharmonies by any of the terms applied to them, because they are in reality nothing and should not be given any kind of name to explain their error meaning. To name a disease tends to give it a place in consciousness; therefore we deny and ignore the name.

Change of Thought

Receptivity to perfect ideas was the absolute requirement that Jesus demanded from those whom He taught and healed. The paralytic who believed he could not walk was healed by Jesus' correct idea about him. Jesus, with His perfect vision of Truth, was able to free the man's body which was bound by nothing but his error thinking. The devil that held the man was the belief that he could not walk. Healing was the result of Jesus' discernment of the truth that man is always free to move. He is a free citizen in a spiritual universe. We do not walk with our legs; we walk with our minds.

Disease is the result of our own limited thought. The mind (soul) is the only life of the body, and the only enduring thing in human nature.

One physician has noted that no one ever dies of what is called disease; he only enters the state of death when his mind loses hold upon the organic structure, and the soul relaxes its grasp upon the body. The body is kept alive by the buoyancy of the mind. When the connection between the mental man and the physical man is severed, then the body dies. We must change our thoughts in order to change the condition of our bodies.

Life Is Ageless

Spirit is eternal and everlasting; it has no age and it does not age. The soul is in a state of constant growth and unfoldment; it continually expands and develops; it never becomes full and finished. The human condition of "old age" is a myth.

As a race we have for ages been deprived in our consciousness of union with our creative source, and the result has been a gradual decrease in vitality until the body has lost the ability to hold its atoms together and consequently has disintegrated. Thus death has come to be accepted as in some mysterious way a part of the divine plan. However, certain biological experiments with cells prove them to be possessed of an ability to reproduce themselves, which at least hints at physical immortality. In the true thought of life, years have no power to take from life that which God has given it. Years have no power to steal from that which God has ordained shall be endless, permanent, enduring, eternal life. "He who believes in the Son has eternal life." "I came that they may have life, and may have it abundantly."

The race mind introduces into the consciousness the thought of age, unless we rise out of it by an understanding of the unchanging life of Christ within us. The age belief says that at a certain period the body begins to grow a little sluggish, to take on flesh, and to be less alive. The cell structures respond to this error belief, the person becomes tired easily, and the body slows down or suffers from pains. All this is of mental origin.

We limit ourselves by dwelling on the thought of death. There is no death or old age—the life in a person of eighty years is exactly the same as the life in a person of five years. We must stop thinking of life as a journey between two points on an endless highway. It is this subconscious feeling that leads to hurry and tension and to the stress that restricts the flow of the vital forces through our body temples. Life is eternal, and we are alive in eternity now. Immortality is not something that occurs after physical passing, but a state of consciousness now. Immortality and eternity are actually the new dimensions of life. In this eternity domain, i.e., in Divine Mind, concurrent with his manifest experience, man is perfect beyond his imperfection, whole beyond his sickness, intelligent beyond his ignorance. In God, in Truth, in the kingdom of heaven, health, wealth, harmony, and peace are constant, and they are now. They are ours to the degree that we can open our eyes to see them, sharpen our faith to believe them, and call forth the will to accept and use them.

Each of us can have all the vibrant and vital life of God that he can accept and use. So-called aging is not the deterioration of life, but the deterioration of our faith, our enthusiasm, our will to progress.

Life is Growth

You don't grow old. When you cease to grow, you are old. The law of life is growth, not aging. Actually, a longer life increases the opportunity for depth in living. In our advanced years, we are capable of being even stronger, happier, healthier than in our youth, and yet we accept the idea of old age and cut our energies off. We do not do things that keep us active and happy because we think we are "too old." We are not at all happy about this development, and it is with resentment, fear, and despondency that we come to grips with the matter of age. But in thought and deed we anticipate, forecast, and decree the very results we bemoan. Age can be a burden and a form of bondage, but it need not be. We are always young enough to express the God-given qualities of life, love, joy, and enthusiasm, and when we are expressing ourself in this way we are unfolding the life of God, which knows no limit. We should forget about the passage of time as a measure. If we had no way to mark time, we would not grow old.

It has been said, "Growing old is no more than a bad habit which a busy man has no time to form." Most people are too careful to "act their age" and as a consequence limit their behavior. Man is an eternal being and is in the midst of eternal life right now.

The number of years we live is unimportant. The kind of years we live is all-important. We have thought only of the dimension of length of years, but we need to consider the dimension of depth. Eternal life is a quality of life; it does not stand for quantity, and any man may have it, no matter what his age in years. A man of eighty may be young, a man of forty old, according to his attitude toward life and living. A man's age is actually none of his business. His spiritual unfoldment and his creative achievements are his business, and happy and youthful is the man who minds his own business.

Life does not, cannot, grow old. We may insist that our strength does diminish and our abilities decline, and that even our health becomes less stable with advancing years. This process is illogical and not God's will, but is merely the product of our own expectancy and error thinking. The God-life that is flowing through us at eighty is the same life that animated, energized, and sustained us in infancy, at eighteen, and at thirty. Life does not get old and weak. Life is eternally vital and vibrant. Life is the perpetual flowing forth into visibility of the illimitable energy of Spirit, and we can have as much as we will claim.

Live in God

We cannot promise good results from prayer when the individual is deliberately living contrary to the spiritual law of life and health. Youth and the good looks of youth are the fruits of young, eager, joyous, and loving attitudes of mind and heart. The flesh pictures forth the fixed attitudes of mind.

Let go of the mental attitude that causes a sense of burden—the belief in age that weights one down with "years." You live in God, not in years; in deeds, not in figures upon a dial. Instead of thinking "I'm getting up in years," get into the spirit of joy in living and loving.

Physical changes may contribute to your sensation of aging. One who does not understand that the body requires certain definite care day by day fails often to do that which is truly best for the body. It is a common error among us that we do not exercise, rest, work, eat, and drink as we should. Healing will come through taking the right mental attitude about the body, then following up this treatment daily with really sensible living habits.

Question Helps

1. "Disease is a condition of consciousness." Explain.

97

2. When seeking a healing, why should one take care not to mention the apparent disorder?
3. How is disease the result of limited thought?
4. When does the body die?
5. Why is the human condition of "old age" a myth?
6. What is the law of life?

Personal Notes

The Way to Healing

All healing methods consist in establishing the unity of the individual and the universal consciousness. The first move in all healing is a recognition on the part of the healer and on the part of the patient that God is present as all-powerful Mind, equal to the healing of every disease, no matter how bad it may appear. The best way to establish unity with the Father-Mind is through prayer to the Father *within*. When you have stilled the outer senses and have become quiet, you are in the mental realm where thoughts are obedient to the word. Error thoughts must be told to go, and true thoughts must be called to take their proper place. Deny the mental cause first, then the physical appearance. For example, nervousness is produced by worry, anxiety, and the like. These mental conditions should be healed first; then the secondary state which they have produced in the body must be denied and dissolved, and the perfect condition affirmed.

In metaphysical treatment we relieve the mind of those thoughts which are antagonistic to Truth. We arrive at a place where we seem to cease individual thinking and just let the Truth of Christ work through us. In the mind of Christ, man exists perfect and whole, regardless of the extent to which the individual accepts disease and outpictures it upon his body. He can be healed to the extent that he will let Christ work. He must be able to behold in his mind's eye this work of purification, redemption, and perfection.

Seeing Christ Perfection

Deny the appearance of disease or discord of any kind, and realize that it is *nothing*. Think of it as dissolved into nothingness, and with your eye of faith see Christ perfection established in the place that needs to manifest the reality of good.

Withdraw the error, then build in the good. Use both denial and affirmation. Do not dwell on the details of negative conditions, for then you give them strength. Do not ask yourself, "What is wrong with me?" for then you are looking at what is wrong, not at what is right. With our spiritual eyes of faith that beholds only the divine image and likeness, we are seeing ourselves as the Father created us in the beginning—whole, illumined, full of faith, perfect. It is not well to dwell upon causes of inharmony, since what we think about, even by way of persistant denials and resistance, becomes more and more a part of our consciousness and hence our experience. Deny the inharmony, then turn immediately to the good you are seeking. Affirm that you are a child of God, perfect and whole as He is perfect and whole.

Denial is a putting away of mental error and an entering into conscious relaxation of both mind and body. To deny what is obvious seems to the intellect ridiculous. In a certain way, such denial is ridiculous, for although on their own plane negative results may be as actual as positive results, negation is not real in final and ultimate Truth. There it has no existence at all. It is like a shadow that has the semblance of life and truth on a plane of shadows but is seen to be unreal in a higher realm of space. Do not therefore resist evil or the sense of reality that it impresses upon the intellect, the body, or human affairs. Instead affirm what is so easily understandable—the great power of God.

Healing Power

In meeting some need for healing with the aid of practical Christianity, though your first object may be simply to be free of a handicap, you have the opportunity of finding something much greater. To know the power that heals is far more important than making your demonstration of healing. By centering your attention on the healing power rather than on the physical need, you will not only achieve the answer to your need but will also gain an understanding of Truth. The basic rules for healing, either for self or for others, are as follows:

Do not be afraid.

Do not judge by appearances.

Look to the healing rather than to the condition.

Know that God can and will heal.

Expect the healing.

We cannot make the law work, but by knowing it will work we can make it easier. All healing is spiritual; all healing comes from God. Jesus emphasized again and again that our part in healing is faith, belief, receptivity. The way to increased faith, belief, and receptivity is through prayer. Prayer opens us up to receive the life that's always there. There is no one method for effective praying, for prayer is not a form but a force. Certain guidelines may help:

1) Relax. Get comfortable and establish yourself in God's presence.

2) Deny all belief in disease and negation of any kind. "There is no disease." "There is no pain."

3) Affim the truth of your perfection, the reality of God. "There is only the life of God flowing freely through me, cleansing, purifying, healing, vitalizing, renewing, restoring me." Identify yourself with the healing life force; know that God is within you.

4) Realization—the incorporation into your being of God Himself, the inner knowing of that Presence. You come to realize that God has heard your prayer; your faith is justified and renewed.

5) Give thanks. Give yourself over to God and let go of the pettyness of small concerns. Praise the Father for all He is.

Unity with God

Sometimes we pray to a God outside of ourselves. It is the God in the midst of us that frees and heals. With our eyes of faith we must see God in our flesh, see wholeness in every part of the body temple. Positive declaration of the truth of one's unity with God sets up a new current of thought power which delivers one from the old beliefs and their depression. When the soul is lifted up and becomes positive, body and affairs are readily healed.

It is not enough to pray. Prayer is one step that you take, but you need other steps. You need to think of God, the all-powerful Healer, as being already within you, in every part of your mind, heart, and body. To keep declaring love and power and life and substance, and yet unconsciously assuming limitations, will cause explosions and congestion that work out in the physical. We need to harmonize our thinking and our prayers with actual living experiences.

Know that God is life, abundant, unfailing, omnipresent, eternal.

Make conscious connection with God life by declaring oneness with it.

Express that oneness in inspired activity.

Work to heal the whole man, for body and consciousness are inseparable. Emphasize wholeness in your affirmations. Healing is a mind process, but to effect permanent healing we must also do the practical physical things to take care of our bodies. We keep it clean inside and out, we get enough exercise, right foods and liquids, proper sleep and relaxation. We are careful about our thoughts, our emotions, our words. We think health, we speak health, we react emotionally in a healthy way. We are careful not to hold any grudges, resentments, or hates. We keep our conscious and subconscious minds packed with healthful ideas. Even if everyone in the room is talking sickness, we do not join in. We silently bless everyone and know that anyone anywhere can be healed. We stand firm on our faith, for however long we need.

If you are subject to some disorder such as a head cold, go in thought to the congested area and repeat quietly: "Peace. The love of God is at work here. My life forces are peaceful and harmonious. There is no resistance in me against the Spirit of God's pure, peaceful life." Quietly and lovingly attract the attention of your disturbed cells and impress upon them the truth that they are a part of the expression of God's harmonious life. Think of the free-flowing life of God being equalized throughout your entire body, doing away with all congestion. Practice harmonious thinking; establish peace both within yourself and among your associates.

Joyful Heart

A joyful, carefree heart is one of the most valuable assets in demonstrating health and wholeness. Exalted joy is linked with gratitude and praise, and it is the consciousness abounding in gratitude and praise that relates us to God and awakens us to the creative impulses of Divine Mind. Joy stimulates naturally the currents of life in the body. Happiness and health are inexorably joined. When you feel good you sing, and a joyous song gets the life circulating in the body. The Spirit of health is always at hand awaiting an opportunity to make whole and to harmonize all discords in the body. Back of every true song is a thought of joy. It is that thought which counts in the end, because it is the thought that invites the healing Spirit. The singing itself restores harmony to tense nerves. Dwelling upon God and cultivating spiritual thoughts stirs one to sing and sets every cell into action, and vibrations are set up to break all crystallized conditions not only in the body but also in the surrounding thought atmosphere. Speaking sets up this vibration within body cells, and singing does this to an even greater extent. This is a creative law that everyone should know, and that everyone can use.

"A cheerful heart is a good medicine." Laughter provides both physical and mental release. It counteracts rigidity and gives one a release from difficulties that weigh on the mind. Its physical benefits are in the expansion of the lungs and the activation of the heart. Laughter has a distinct social value in making a person congenial and responsive. Lastly, it has an effect on the emotions, providing an emotional release that makes for a wholesome and cheerful outlook. Often when joy enters the mind, the grip on an adverse condition is released.

All healing systems recognize joy as a beneficent factor in the restoration of health to the sick. The mind puts kinks in the nerves. A fear thought can stop the life flow through the body, causing congestion. An impact of energy, such as physical exercise, electricity, or a joyous shock is necessary to break up fear congestion. Ease the fear, which is mental cause, and the problem will be no more. The most effective and direct way to deal with fear is by laughing.

We can find healing by changing our thoughts about our bodies, by blessing and praising the life and intelligence in every part. You can praise and bless your way out of every negative condition of mind or body. So if you find it difficult at first to quit thinking or talking in terms of illness or disease, begin to add the idea of blessing to your thoughts and words. When there are aches and pains, then is the time to praise your body even more for the good work that it is doing, for the life and intelligence that are in every part. Commend your splendid body for its marvelous construction and its perfect work. You can praise a weak body into strength; a fearful heart into peace and trust; shattered nerves into poise and power; a failing business into prosperity and success; want and insufficiency into supply and support.

Give thanks even *before* you have manifested receipt of something. "Whatever you ask in prayer, believe that you receive it, and you will." Giving thanks in advance brings about what you want. Praise and thanksgiving release Spirit energy that has been pent up, unused, in the cells. It releases the energy to be put into action by creative Mind. Thoughts of praise and thanksgiving carry life, intelligence, and substance to that which is praised, invigorating and renewing it.

The Exercise of Faith

Jesus demanded faith on the part of those whom He healed, and with that faith as the point of mental and spiritual contact, He released the latent energy in the atomic structure of His patients and they were restored to life and health. He knew that the blessing of health comes through the exercise of faith on the part of the man who seeks it, that faith opens the mind to the inflow of power from on high, and that the power of the Highest heals all disease of soul and body.

When faith is sufficiently strong to dissolve all adverse conditions and to open the mind fully to the power of God, healing is instantaneous. Faith on our part transforms innate desire and will into an active force, a vitalizing, healing power. We no longer just feel in a vague way that we should be well and strong; we put ourselves actively into this belief and stand by our faith. We take our stand for healing and know we will be healed. We choose to live. We do not wonder any longer if it is God's will for us to be healed. We do not try to make sickness into a virtue. We turn away from belief in sickness or disease, from the belief that we cannot be healed, and make our every thought and word an affirmation of life. This is faith in action—to believe in God, to believe in life, to believe in healing, and to keep on believing.

Faith is the confidence of the mind that invisible substance is the source of visible material things. "Faith is the assurance of things hoped for, the conviction of things not seen." Faith enables man to see through the shadowy forms of false concepts—the creations of the natural man—and to behold the real. God lives in each heart, and he who consciously dwells in His presence comes into an understanding of the creative powers of the universe. Into this "secret place of the Most High" no thought of disease or destruction can enter. Here the healing, soothing balm of divine faith pours itself out, seeking to expand and to enliven God's perfection in the whole consciousness. It is the constant mingling and intermingling of the conscious intelligence with faith that establishes the healing consciousness in man.

Faith in its highest form is an exalted idea, and the most exalted idea that man can have is that he is spiritual, that he is related directly to the one great Spirit, and that through Spirit he can do mighty works through faith. *Anything* can be accomplished through faith. Doctors have found that they need not use real drugs, if they have the confidence of the patient. Anyone can lift himself out of the physical plane and heal all his ills by cultivating his faith in God through affirmation of his spiritual power. The capacity of the mind that enables it to make contact with the realm of creative ideas is faith, and faith is superenthusiasm. You must have such confidence in your ability to make union with creative Mind that you fuse the two. "Whoever . . . does not doubt in his heart, but believes that what he says will come to pass, it will be done for him." Here in a nutshell Jesus has stated the law and its fulfillment. The one and only reason that we do not always succeed in our demonstrations is that we do not persist in our mental work.

Alive with Faith

Is this a time of illness for you? This then is the time for faith! It is the time for remembering that your body is the temple of the living God, that the cells of your body are imbued with living substance, that the healing power of God is mighty in the midst of you. "With God all things are possible." When you proclaim your faith in God as life you feel the strength of this faith, for the faith in you is God-inspired and grows as you express and use it.

106

In the face of illness or disease, proclaim your faith. Bless your body in the realization that every cell in it is alight and aglow with healing life. Declare your faith in the one life, God-life, in the one power, God-power. Declare your faith in the renewing, rebuilding, restoring process of life that is now perfecting and healing you in every part.

When Peter tried to walk on the water to meet Jesus, he went down in the sea of doubt. He saw too much wetness in the water. He saw the negative side of the proposition, and it weakened his demonstration. If you want to demonstrate, never consider the negative side. If mountains seem to oppose the carrying out of your plans, say with Napoleon that there shall be no Alps. The man who is grounded in faith does not measure his thoughts or his acts by the world's standard of facts. Those who are in spiritual understanding know that certain things do exist in Spirit and become substantial and real to the one who dwells, thinks, and lives in faith.

We must hold steadily to our faith in order for it to be able to accomplish its purposes. Many have learned how to hold the truth about health in the midst of most adverse appearances, and they clearly understand that they are not telling falsehoods when they deny sickness right in the face of its appearance. Deny ill temper, vanity, greed, selfishness; affirm the unselfishness, purity, uprightness, and integrity of the higher self. Persons who are quickened spiritually can do very much greater works through the law of faith than those who are caught in the material consciousness.

Question Helps

1. What is the best way to establish unity with Father-Mind?
2. Discuss the use of denials and affirmations in healing.

3. What are basic rules for healing? List the guidelines for effective prayer.
4. What is the most effective and direct way to deal with fear?
5. Why is it necessary to exercise faith in order to be healed?
6. "A time of illness is a time of faith." Explain.

Personal Notes

Treatments for Specific Disorders

Mental causes are so complex that it is impossible to point out in all cases the specific thought that causes a certain disease, but there are basic mind functions, and when one is affected it in turn affects all the others. Nearly all sick people lack vital force, hence a life treatment is good for all. A favorite affirmation is "I fairly sizzle with zeal and enthusiasm and spring forth with a mighty faith to do the things that ought to be done by me." Hate, anger, jealousy, malice, and the like are almost universal in human consciousness, and a treatment for love will prove a healing balm for all. Fear of poverty burdens most people, and the prosperity treatment will be effective in relieving the symptoms brought on by this fear. Remember that the objective of all treatment is to raise the mind to the Christ consciousness, through which all true healing is accomplished.

Relax

The prevailing ills of the abdominal region—constipation, tumors, and the like—are caused by constriction of the whole body energy. The faculties centering in the head are responsible for this slowing down of the life forces. The will, operating through the front brain, controls the circulation of the life force in the whole organism. A tense will, set to accomplish some personal end, keys everything to that end and puts a limitation on the activity of every other function. Persons who try too hard to have their own way cause a rigidity and tension in their bodies. This impedes the free action of the heart, and circulation becomes irregular. The set determination to succeed in some chosen field of action, study, profession, business, or personal ambition calls most of the body energy to the head and starves the other centers. Relax, and let God guide you: "Not my will, but thine, be done."

Cultivate Peace

The action of the stomach is governed by a nerve center called the solar plexus, which is in close touch with the thinking center in the head. If a man's thoughts are excitedly or inharmoniously active, the orderly process of digestion becomes disturbed. The spiritual remedy is to cultivate a peaceful, trustful state of mind. Eat in a leisurely manner and dispel worldly cares from your mind.

Some persons have a habit of saying that certain foods do not agree with them. The fact very often is that they disagree in their mind with the food, and that causes the food to seem to disagree with them. They should see that their food is really good and nourishing and then agree with it, and so become willing to eat the good of the land thankfully and fearlessly. Good food does not affect the stomach, but adverse, contrary thoughts do.

A good tonic for the stomach is to look on the bright side of everything. Regardless of apparent error, keep your thought and word praising and rejoicing. When you have sweetened all the secretions of your body with joy and praise, you will have changed the chemistry of your whole organism.

The nerve center from which the eliminative function directs the emptying of the intestines is located deep in the lower bowels. This center is very sensitive to thoughts about substance and all materiality. A gripping mental hold on material things will cause constipation. A relaxation of the mind and a loosening of the grip on material possessions will bring about freedom in bowel action.

The Order of Harmony

An affirmative thought sometimes produces a congested condition throughout the body and interferes

110

with elimination. Continued strenuous affirmations, even of Truth, will sometimes cause constipation. The remedy is to relax, to let go. The words of Truth that you have affirmed must have time to work out in the subconsciousness. We must free ourselves to express the wisdom and power of Spirit. The passing away of the old and the incoming of the new are results of the outworking of the law, and man should assist in bringing about these changes. Let go all weariness, doubt, and fear. The healing power is active throughout your whole being, with all its cleansing, discriminating, purifying effects. Work with it, not against it.

On the other hand, where the "no" phase of mind, that is, the use of denial, is too much in evidence, the whole consciousness is in relaxation. This excessive negation makes the thought indefinite and vacillating, the body weak and flabby. This may also lead to looseness of the bowels, a loss of substance. This can be healed by a treatment to induce courage and fearlessness.

The nerves, being a manifestation of mind, respond to the thoughts of the mind that are sent along them. Therefore, in order that the nerves may remain strong and peaceful, one's thoughts must be harmonious, kindly, and true. Aches and pains in the head usually imply a need for the better functioning of some organ of the body or for more health and harmony in the nerves. The head is likely to suffer in sympathy with any part of the system that is out of order. Affirm life, love, peace, and health in every part of the body. Deny all tenseness; relax.

Worried, anxious thoughts cause congestion in the head. To heal a cold, relax and affirm harmony throughout the body. Deny the power of mortal thought to interfere in the perfect order of the body. Deny the thought that you can take a cold; your lot is perfect health in all parts. Do not do too much material thinking. Center on Truth, but do not hold your true thoughts all in your head. Realize the vitalizing power of Spirit all through your body.

Singlemindedness

Greater fearlessness, love, and uprightness of mind are necessary for the healing of the heart. In order that fear may be eliminated, purity of heart must be established and divine love must be quickened in the consciousness. To be "pure in heart" means to be of one purpose, one aim. That one purpose should be to give God first place in your life and to work to express Him always. This singlemindedness will make every part of the body whole, and the heart will respond with every other body function.

Intemperance

Intemperance, both of eating and drinking, has a cause lying deeper than appetite. It is evidence that the soul is yearning for something; the outer craving indicates the inner lack. Recognition of this true need and affirmation of the filling substance of God's love reduces this craving. As repeated affirmations of life and love stimulate the life essence within the body, the desire for outside stimulants will cease.

There is a tendency to put on weight as one begins to realize and demonstrate prosperity, especially when prosperity is linked to the accumulation of material objects. This indicates too much thought about getting and too little about giving. To heal this condition, establish a balance of giving and receiving. Deny accumulation; affirm the free flow of God's good through you. Deny belief in materiality; affirm true spiritual substance.

Just and Wise Life

The liver seems to be linked with the function of mental discrimination. Harsh judgments of others often lead to a disorder of the liver. Condemnation in any of its forms retards freedom of action in the discriminative faculty. When we hold ourselves in guilt and condemnation, the natural energies of the mind are weakened and the whole body becomes inert. Affirm the universal justice of Spirit. We cannot always discern it at work, but it overrides all injustice if we will believe and affirm it.

Strength and purity are the central thoughts for the establishment of abiding health in the kidneys.

To heal anemia, which is a seeming deficiency in the blood, a greater realization of the strength and substance of life is needed. Affirm life.

To heal high blood pressure, release all tension. *Consciously* relax. Heal stiff joints by freeing all tension from nerves, muscles, tendons, and joints.

In the healing of cuts, bruises, or burns, first realize the omnipresence of Spirit, wholeness, health, peace, and harmony. Affirm free-flowing Christ love and life throughout the body.

Love Softens and Heals

Love will soften and heal any hard condition in mind or body, such as hardening of the arteries or arthritis. The love of Jesus Christ heals by freeing the mind from the many worries, fears, and other errors that tend to impede digestion, assimilation, or elimination. Affirm thoughts of love and good will toward everyone and everything. Feel yourself filled to overflowing with love.

Vision of Truth

The eye represents the discerning capacity of the mind. It is the physical organ that is the outpicturing of the ability of the mind to discern, mentally, physically, spiritually, all that is. Seeing is a mental process, and the eyes are the instruments that register what the mind has been trained to think and to behold. When our mental processes are in perfectly harmonious accord with the ideas of Divine Mind, our sight is perfect and our eyes function properly, with nothing coming between to hinder.

To heal the eyes, declare that your perception of spiritual Truth is clear and strong and that your faith in the power of the formless and invisible is unshaken. Affirm God as the discerning power of your life. Realize that sight is not material but spiritual. To cure astigmatism, nearsightedness, or farsightedness, set your ideas right. Place your inner vision of Truth in the right focus, and your eyes will respond with true vision.

Receptive to Spirit

The ear represents the receptive capacity of the mind. It is the instrument of the mind through which we receive instruction from God's mind. Only as a person is open and receptive to the voice from within and willing to be guided in all ways by this voice is his hearing sense lifted to the spiritual plane and put to the use God ordained it should have. Listening within for the still, small voice with a mind consecrated to obedience trains the ears to their true function. To heal the ear, open the mind to receive Truth. Man hears with his mind rather than with his ears. If this mind is so occupied with its own preconceived thoughts that it is slow to grasp ideas conveyed to it by the higher self within or by persons without, dullness of hearing often manifests itself. Affirm openness and receptiveness; deny personal will and solidified opinion. Practice at listening within.

The nose represents the detective and initiative capacities of the mind. The tongue represents the judging capacity of the mind and serves to discriminate among the appropriate correct input for the body organism. Feeling represents the loving capacity of the

114

mind. Intuition is the natural knowing capacity of the mind.

All the senses are built to enable the mind to function in its capacity to find that which is good for the soul and body and to direct the body toward the appropriation of it. The mind that is in tune with the true being, the Christ self, is constantly using its physical tools, the senses, to nourish, guide, and protect the body temple.

Question Helps

1. What is the objective of all healing treatments?
2. Why is it important to keep harmonious thoughts?
3. What does it mean to be "pure in heart"?
4. Explain what is meant by mental discrimination.
5. How does love heal?
6. "Man hears with his mind rather than his ears." Explain.

Personal Notes

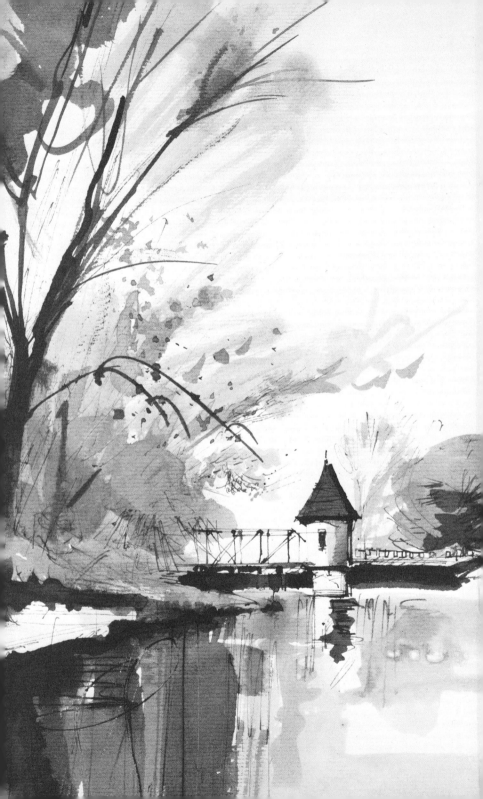

Two Healing Testimonies

The manifestation of a perfect body is within the reach of each and every human being alive today. Healings that amaze and baffle physicians are taking place every day through the power and strength of persons who know God as the source of their perfect health. Charles and Myrtle Fillmore, cofounders of the Unity movement, were well aware of the innate perfection of their own bodies and of the unlimited power they possessed to manifest that perfection. Charles' own words best tell his story:

"I can testify to my own healing of tuberculosis of the hip. When a boy of ten I was taken with what was at first diagnosed as rheumatism but developed into a very serious case of hip disease. I was in bed over a year, and from that time an invalid in constant pain for twenty-five years, or until I began the application of the divine law. Two very large tubercular abcesses developed at the head of the hip bone, which the doctors said would finally drain away my life. But I managed to get about on crutches, with a four-inch cork-and-steel extension on the right leg. The hip bone was out of the socket and stiff. The leg shriveled and ceased to grow. The whole right side became involved; my right ear was deaf and my right eye weak. From hip to knee the flesh was a glassy adhesion with but little sensation.

"When I began applying the spiritual treatment there was for a long time slight response in the leg, but I felt better, and I found that I began to hear with the right ear. Then gradually I noticed that I had more feeling in the leg. Then as the years went by the ossified joint began to get limber, and the shrunken flesh filled out until the right leg was almost equal to the other. Then I discarded the cork-and-steel extension and wore *an ordinary shoe with a double heel about an inch in height. Now the leg is almost as large as the other, the muscles are restored, and although the hip bone is not yet in the socket, I am certain that it soon will be and that I shall be made perfectly whole. . . .*

"I have watched the restoration year after year as I applied the power of thought, and I know it is under divine law. So I am satisfied that here is proof of a law that the mind builds the body and can restore it."

Myrtle has written the story of her healing this way:

"I myself was once an emaciated little woman, upon whom relatives and doctors had placed the stamp 'T.B.' [tuberculosis]. And this was only one of the ailments— there were others considered beyond any help, except possibly the changing of structures through an operation. There were family problems too. We were a sickly lot, and came to the place where we were unable to provide for our children. In the midst of all this gloom, we kept looking for the way out, which we felt sure would be revealed. It was! The light of God revealed to us—the thought came to me first—that life was of God, that we were inseparably one with the source, and that we inherited from the divine and perfect Father. What that revelation did to me at first was not apparent to the senses. But it held my mind up above the negation, and I began to claim my birthright and to act as though I believed myself the child of God, filled with His life. I gained. And others saw that there was something new in me.

"I knew that God, whom I could call Father, would not create imperfect children. As I thought of it, I began to realize that I was truly God's child, and that because of this I must of necessity inherit from Him. Then . . . I saw that the life that is in us is the life of God. Therefore, I reasoned, the plan of God must be an inherent part of the mind of man. . . . I began to live with God, and to talk with Him. . . .

"God revealed to me that my body was intelligent; that I could direct and praise it, and it would respond.... He was giving me His life, substance, and intelligence, and I was to use them, even more freely than I had used the blessings my Earthly father had given me.

"I told the life in my liver that it was not torpid or inert, but full of vigor and energy. I told the life in my stomach that it was not weak or inefficient, but energetic, strong, and intelligent. I told the life in my abdomen that it was no longer infested with ignorant ideas of disease, put there by myself and by doctors, but that it was all athrill with the sweet, pure, wholesome energy of God. I told my limbs that they were active and strong. I told my eyes that they did not see of themselves but that they expressed the sight of Spirit, and that they were drawing on an unlimited source. I told them that they were young eyes, clear, bright eyes, because the light of God shone right through them. I told my heart that the pure love of Jesus Christ flowed in and out through its beatings and that all the world felt its joyous pulsation.

"I went to all the life centers of my body and spoke words of Truth to them—words of strength and power. I asked their forgiveness for the foolish, ignorant course that I had pursued in the past, when I condemned them and called them weak, inefficient, and diseased. I did not become discouraged at their being slow to wake up, but kept right on, both silently and aloud, declaring the words of Truth, until the organs responded. And neither did I forget to tell them that they were free, unlimited Spirit. I told them ... that they were not corruptible flesh, but centers of life and energy omnipresent....

"I promised [the Father] that I would never, never again retard the free flow of that life through my mind and my body by any false word or thought; that I would always bless it and encourage it with true thoughts and words in its wise work of building up my body temple;

that I would use all diligence and wisdom in telling it just what I wanted it to do.

"I also saw that I was using the life of the Father in thinking thoughts and speaking words, and I became very watchful as to what I thought and said.

"I did not let any worried or anxious thoughts into my mind, and I stopped speaking gossipy, frivolous, petulant, angry words.

"You ask what restored me to vigorous health. It was a change of mind from the old, carnal mind that believes in sickness to the Christ Mind of life and permanent health. 'Be ye transformed by the renewing of your mind.' 'As he thinketh within himself, so is he.' I applied spiritual laws effectively, blessing my body temple until it manifested the innate health of Spirit. These wonderful laws will work for you too when you apply them diligently and in faith."

References

Butterworth, Eric *Life Is for Living*
Cady, H. Emilie *God a Present Help*
Cady, H. Emilie *Lessons in Truth*
Fillmore, Charles *Atom-Smashing Power of Mind*
Fillmore, Charles *Christian Healing*
Fillmore, Charles *Dynamics for Living*
Fillmore, Charles *Jesus Christ Heals*
Fillmore, Charles *The Twelve Powers of Man*
Fillmore, Charles & Cora *Teach Us to Pray*
Fillmore, Cora Dedrick *Christ Enthroned in Man*
Fillmore, Lowell *Health, Wealth, and Happiness*
Fillmore, Lowell *Things to Be Remembered*
Myrtle Fillmore's Healing Letters
Fillmore, Myrtle *How to Let God Help You*
Lynch, Richard *Health and Spiritual Healing*
Lynch, Richard *Know Thyself*
MacDougall, Mary Katherine *Healing Now*
Schobert, Theodosia DeWitt *Divine Remedies*
Shanklin, Imelda *Selected Studies*
Smock, Martha *Halfway Up the Mountain*
Smock, Martha *Meet It with Faith*
Whitney, Frank B. *Be of Good Courage*
Whitney, Frank B. *Mightier Than Circumstance*
Wilson, Ernest C. *The Emerging Self*
Wilson, Ernest C. *The Great Physician*

Additional Notes